Study Guide

Health Psychology
An Introduction to Behavior and Health

SEVENTH EDITION

Linda Brannon
McNeese State University

Jess Feist
McNeese State University

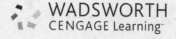
Prepared by

Linda Brannon
McNeese State University

Jess Feist
McNeese State University

WADSWORTH
CENGAGE Learning

Australia • Brazil • Japan • Korea • Mexico • Singapore • Spain • United Kingdom • United States

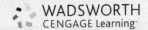
ISBN-13: 978-0-495-60348-1
ISBN-10: 0-495-60348-1

Wadsworth
10 Davis Drive
Belmont, CA 94002-3098
USA

Cengage Learning is a leading provider of customized learning solutions with office locations around the globe, including Singapore, the United Kingdom, Australia, Mexico, Brazil, and Japan. Locate your local office at:
international.cengage.com/region

Cengage Learning products are represented in Canada by Nelson Education, Ltd.

For your course and learning solutions, visit
academic.cengage.com

Purchase any of our products at your local college store or at our preferred online store
www.ichapters.com

Printed in the United States of America
2 3 4 5 6 7 8 13 12 11 10

Table of Contents

Preface

To Students—

We have designed this Study Guide to accompany our *Health Psychology: Introduction to Behavior and Health* (7th ed.), with each chapter corresponding to a chapter in that text. Each of the 16 chapters of the Study Guide is divided as follows:

- **Learning Objectives** appear at the beginning of each chapter to provide an overview of what you should learn from each chapter.

- **Fill in the Rest of the Story** is a fill-in-the-blanks exercise that tests your ability to recall important terms, concepts, and definitions. Fill in the blanks and check your answers with those provided at the end of the chapter.

- **Multiple Choice Questions** allow you to test your recognition memory. Many of these items may be similar to those you will see on your quizzes and tests. Mark your answers and check their accuracy.

- **Matching Exercises** are oriented toward helping you connect important elements that may be confusing, such as concepts and their definitions, researchers and their research, and theories and their main points.

- Defining **Key Terms** is another type of study aid. Grasping these important terms and putting them into your own words may help you integrate this information, recognize, and discuss it.

- **Visual Exercises** appear in some of the chapters and will challenge you to identify important information visually. These exercises are similar to figures in the text, and you should complete the figure by supplying missing labels, and then check the text for the correct answers.

- **Essay Questions** measure your ability to organize and present key points in each chapter. We have provided an extensive answer outline for each essay question to allow you to check not only information but also organization.

- **Let's Get Personal** is an individualized exercise that gives you an opportunity to integrate the health information in each chapter into your own life.

Purchasing the textbook and study guide are only a preliminary step toward mastering the course material in health psychology. Unfortunately, we have discovered no magical way to make studying effortless. We designed the exercises in this study guide to give you a variety of approaches to learn health psychology, but none of these study devices will help if you do not use them. Reading the text and attending class are important in learning and in making good grades. We hope that you use this study guide to organize and assimilate the volume of information in health psychology. We believe that working through the study guide exercises can help you make better grades and can make health psychology part of your life.

Good luck in studying health psychology,

Linda Brannon

Linda Brannon

Jess Feist

Jess Feist

CHAPTER 1
Introducing Health Psychology

Learning Objectives

After studying Chapter 1, you should be able to

1. Describe the changes in patterns of disease that occurred during the 20th century.

2. Trace the changes in the health care system that have resulted in escalating cost.

3. Compare the biomedical model and the biopsychosocial model of health.

4. Discuss psychology's involvement in the field of health care.

5. Describe the training and work of health psychology practitioners and contrast that training and work with that of health psychology researchers.

Fill in the Rest of the Story

I. The Changing Field of Health

During the 20th century, the field of health changed because patterns of illness changed. In 1900, most illnesses were _____ and of short duration, and now most are _____ and relate to behavior and lifestyle.

A. Patterns of Disease and Death

Currently, the two leading causes of death in the United States and other industrialized countries are _____ and _____. These two diseases affect older people more often than young people. Teenagers and young adults are most likely to die of _____ _____. Ethnic background is also a factor in life expectancy, but poverty and _____ level relate to ethnic background, making this factor difficult to determine. During the 20th century, life expectancy has grown from about 47 years in 1900 to more than 77 years in 2005, and most of that gain has been due to a decrease in _____ _____.

B. Escalating Cost of Medical Care

The cost of medical care has risen more rapidly than _____, leading

some people to question the cost effectiveness of cures and to emphasize the role of

_____ in containing medical costs.

C. What Is Health?

The traditional definition of health comes from the biomedical model, which holds that

disease is due to the presence of an outside agent called a pathogen that causes disease. An

alternative model, the _____ model, adds psychological and social

factors to biological ones, resulting in a more comprehensive view of health and illness.

Health psychologists follow this model, which defines health as a _____

state; that is, a state of well being. This definition is compatible with the positive psychology

movement, which emphasizes how factors such as _____ affect health.

II. Psychology's Involvement in Health

Psychology's involvement in health concentrates on _____ factors in the

development of many chronic diseases. Health psychologists also help people cope with stress,

pain, and chronic illness.

A. Psychology in Medical Settings

Until the development of health psychology, psychologists who were involved in medical

training either taught in _____ school or provided clinical consultation.

B. The Contribution of Psychosomatic Medicine

The view that physical illness has its roots in psychological and emotional conflicts is

called _____ medicine. This movement exerted a _____

influence in drawing attention to the connection between emotion and disease but a

_____ influence in developing the belief that some diseases are "all in

people's heads."

C. The Emergence of Behavioral Medicine

The interdisciplinary field of _____ _____ attempts to integrate behavioral and biomedical knowledge and techniques and apply this knowledge to prevention, diagnosis, treatment, and rehabilitation.

D. The Emergence of Health Psychology

Health psychology is that field of psychology dealing with the scientific study of _____ that relate to health enhancement, prevention, and rehabilitation. Psychologists interested in health-related issues founded the psychological specialty of health psychology and formed Division 38 of the _____ _____ Association.

III. The Profession of Health Psychology

Health psychology can contribute to health by accumulating information on factors that relate to health and illness, using its expertise in research and measurement for health matters, and applying the principles of behavior change to eliminate _____ behavior and to incorporate healthy _____ into people's lifestyles.

A. The Training of Health Psychologists

Health psychologists receive a solid core of training at the _____ level before continuing an additional two (or more) years of training in a variety of health-related subjects. The training of clinical health psychologists prepares them for work that is _____ in nature; that is, health psychologists frequently work with a team of health professionals, including physicians, nurses, physical therapists, and counselors..

B. The Work of Health Psychologists

Health psychologists work in a variety of settings and perform many different functions. Health psychologists who work in universities typically teach and conduct _____, whereas clinical health psychologists usually provide _____, diagnosis, and therapy services in hospitals, clinics, HMOs, and private practices.

3

Multiple Choice Questions

_____ 1. Which of these statements is true?
   a. The United States has the highest life expectancy of any nation in the world.
   b. The best definition of good health is the absence of disease.
   c. The increase of life expectancy in the United States during the 20th century was due mostly to better medical and emergency room care.
   d. The increase in life expectancy in the United States during the 20th century was mostly a result of changes in lifestyles.
   e. None of these statements is true.

_____ 2. Which of these has been a major health trend in the Unites States since 1900?
   a. Health has been more frequently defined as the absence of illness.
   b. Acute diseases have replaced chronic diseases as the leading causes of death.
   c. The cost of medical care has risen faster than the rate of inflation.
   d. Population shifts to southern states have lowered illness rates.

_____ 3. In the United States, death rates due to _____ have increased during the last few years of the 20th century and the first few years of the 21st century.
   a. cancer
   b. cardiovascular disease
   c. homicides
   d. all of the above
   e. none of the above

_____ 4. For young people in the United States, the leading cause of death is
   a. unintentional injuries.
   b. suicides.
   c. homicides.
   d. sexual behaviors.

_____ 5. Most deaths in the United States are the result of
   a. acute, infectious diseases.
   b. lack of exercise.
   c. chronic diseases.
   d. sexual behaviors.

_____ 6. In the United States, the leading cause of death for children ages 1 to 5 years old is
   a. heart disease.
   b. HIV infection.
   c. cancer.
   d. unintentional injuries.

_____ 7. Life expectancy in the United States has _____ since 1900.
  a. increased by about 20 years
  b. increased by about 30 years
  c. decreased by about 10 years
  d. remained about the same

_____ 8. In United States, the primary reason for the large increase in life expectancy during the 20th century was
  a. the introduction of more reliable medical equipment.
  b. better training of health care providers.
  c. the large decrease in deaths from cardiovascular diseases.
  d. the decrease in infant mortality.

_____ 9. The biopsychosocial view of health is most likely to be held by
  a. health psychologists.
  b. the federal government.
  c. traditional medicine.
  d. people who see health as an ideal.

_____ 10. Any agent that can cause a disease is called a(n)
  a. risk factor.
  b. illness.
  c. infection.
  d. pathogen.

_____ 11. In the United States, which ethnic group has the most serious health problems?
  a. African Americans
  b. Hispanic Americans
  c. European Americans
  d. Asian Americans

_____ 12. People who have attended college _____ than those who have graduated from high school.
  a. are more likely to smoke cigarettes
  b. are healthier and live longer
  c. are less likely to engage in a program of physical exercise
  d. are less likely to experience chronic diseases but more likely to have acute diseases

_____ 13. Beau attributes his "cold" to not getting enough sleep and to recent stressful life experiences. Thus, it seems that Beau's beliefs are consistent with
  a. the biochemical model of health.
  b. the biomedical model of health.
  c. the biopsychosocial model of health.
  d Cartesian dualism.

_____ 14. That aspect of medicine that views physical illnesses as having emotional and psychological components is called
   a. health psychology.
   b. behavioral health.
   c. Cartesian medicine.
   d. psychosomatic medicine.

_____ 15. Behavioral health emphasizes
   a. the importance of psychosomatic medicine.
   b. the prevention of illness and the enhancement of health.
   c. the treatment of disease.
   d. the importance of stress in chronic illnesses.

_____ 16. The discipline that focuses on the scientific study of those behaviors related to health enhancement, disease prevention, and rehabilitation is called
   a. behavioral health.
   b. psychosomatic medicine.
   c. behavioral medicine.
   d. health psychology.

_____ 17. During the last 25 years of the 20th century, psychology became more involved in people's health mostly by
   a. practicing psychosomatic medicine.
   b. investigating those behaviors that enhance health and prevent disease.
   c. treating mental diseases.
   d. treating physical diseases.

_____ 18. Health psychologists are most involved with
   a. treating acute diseases.
   b. lengthening the span of life.
   c. determining the causes of disease.
   d. decreasing the incidence of psychological disorders.
   e. adding healthy years to people's lives.

_____ 19. Health psychologists are MOST likely to
   a. work as part of an interdisciplinary team.
   b. work as a practitioner in a solo private mental health care practice.
   c. go to medical school after finishing a doctoral degree in psychology.
   d. do all of the above.

Key Terms

Define each of the following:

behavioral medicine —

biopsychosocial model —

chronic diseases —

health psychology —

pathogen —

The Biopsychosocial Model

Fill in the spaces below, listing the psychological, sociological, and biological factors that contribute to health outcomes, then draw in arrows to indicate the types and direction of the interactions in the biopsychosocial model.

Psychology

_____

_____

_____

_____

_____

_____

_____

_____

_____

_____

Biology

_____

_____

_____

_____

_____

_____

Sociology

_____

_____

_____

_____

Outcomes

Health _____

Essay Questions

1. Discuss the role of ethnicity in health and illness. What factors complicate the interpretation of these effects?

2. How do behavioral medicine and health psychology differ? How are they similar?

3. A friend of yours (who is a psychology major but who has not taken health psychology) tells you, "I don't want to be a health psychologist because I don't want to work with sick people in a hospital." Is her assessment correct in its description of the work done by health psychologists?

Let's Get Personal—
What Is Your Definition of Health?

What is your personal definition of health—that is, what does being healthy mean? Write down what a healthy person should be and should be able to do. What types of situations or conditions would prevent a person from being healthy?

Does your definition come closer to the biomedical or the biopsychosocial view of health and illness?

What does being healthy mean to you?

A healthy person should be able to

A person is not healthy if he or she:

Is your view closer to the biomedical or biopsychosocial view?

Answers

Fill in the Rest of the Story

I.   acute (infectious); chronic
I.A. heart disease (cardiovascular disease); cancer; unintentional injuries (accidents); educational (income); infant mortality
I.B. inflation, prevention
I.C. biopsychosocial; positive; optimism (hope)
II.   behavioral (lifestyle)
II.A. medical
II.B. psychosomatic; positive; negative
II.C. behavioral medicine
II.D. behaviors, American Psychological
III. unhealthy; behaviors
III.A. doctoral; collaborative (interdisciplinary)
III.B. research; assessment

Multiple Choice

1.	e	6.	d	11.	a	16.	d
2.	c	7.	b	12.	b	17.	b
3.	e	8.	d	13.	c	18.	e
4.	a	9.	a	14.	d	19.	a
5.	c	10.	d	15.	b		

Good points to include in your essay answers:

1. Ethnicity plays a role in life expectancy.
    A. European Americans have substantially longer life expectancies than African Americans.
    B. The role of ethnicity is not entirely clear because poverty and low socioeconomic status also relate to ethnicity in the United States.
        1. Poverty is related to ethnicity; poor people have restricted access to medical services and lower life expectancy than people with more money.
        2. Low educational level is also related to ethnicity, and less educated people are more likely to exhibit risky health-related behaviors.

2. Behavioral medicine and health psychology have both differences and similarities.
    A. Differences
        1. Behavioral medicine developed as a result of the Yale conference, and health psychology was the result of an APA task force.
        2. Behavioral medicine is an interdisciplinary field; although health psychology has drawn from several fields, it remains within psychology.

3. The professional societies and journals differ for each area.
4. The work of those in behavioral medicine tends to concentrate on diagnosis and treatment, whereas health psychologists may also be involved in prevention.

B. Similarities
1. Both have similar goals, including the integration of biomedical and behavioral knowledge in order to prevent disease and aid in diagnosis and treatment.
2. Both draw from many fields, including medicine, physiology, psychology, and sociology.
3. Both those in health psychology and those in behavioral medicine can join the others' professional societies and consider the others' journals important to their own work.
4. The work of health psychologists who concentrate on people who are already ill may be indistinguishable from the work of those in the field of behavioral medicine.

3. A. Her assessment is true for some, but not for most, health psychologists.
   B. The work setting of some health psychologists is similar to other psychologists.
   1. Like other research psychologists, health psychologists who conduct research usually are employed in educational settings where they combine teaching and research.
   2. Like other clinical or counseling psychologists, health psychologists who provide services may work in private practice, in hospitals or clinics, or in health maintenance organizations (HMOs), where they provide diagnosis and treatment.
   3. Clinical and counseling psychologists provide services to people who have diagnosed mental disorders, making them "sick" in some sense but not in the sense that most people use the word.
   C. Some health psychologists work in medical settings oriented toward providing care for the physically ill.
   1. Some health psychology researchers teach medical students and participate in research as part of biomedical research teams.
   2. Some health psychologists who provide services work as part of teams that provide services to people who are physically sick, either as ancillary treatment or as treatment for the physical disorder.
   3. Health psychologists are more likely to be involved in providing preventive services, but this work involves providing services to people who are not sick.

CHAPTER 2
Conducting Health Research

Learning Objectives

After studying Chapter 2, you should be able to

1. Define placebo and explain how that phenomenon affects both research and treatment.

2. Discuss how psychology research methods apply to the field of health psychology.

3. Discuss how epidemiology research methods apply to the field of health psychology.

4. Explain how researchers establish causal relationships.

5. Evaluate how theory and measurement contribute to health psychology research.

Fill in the Rest of the Story

I. The Placebo in Research and Treatment

A placebo is an inactive substance or condition that can cause people to change and even to

improve their behavior. Both learning and _____, or belief, contribute to this

effect.

A. Treatment and the Placebo

In general, improvements from placebo treatments are about _____ %. Placebos can

also produce negative effects called the _____ effect.

B. Research and the Placebo

Researchers try to control for the placebo effect by using single-blind and _____-

_____ designs.

II. Research Methods in Psychology

Psychologists use a variety of research methods to study human behavior.

A. Correlational Studies

Correlational studies are one type of _____ research. These studies

indicate the degree of relationship between two variables, yielding correlation coefficients that may fall between the values of _____ to _____. However, correlational studies do not demonstrate _____ and effect.

B. Cross-Sectional and Longitudinal Studies

Cross-sectional studies are conducted at one point in time and often compare people of different _____. Studies that follow participants over an extended period of time are _____, which have the advantage of revealing _____ trends.

C. Experimental Designs

Experimental designs allow researchers to demonstrate cause and effect by manipulating the _____ variable and observing its effect on the _____ variable. Researchers using an experimental design must control for participants' expectation that treatment will be effective regardless of actual effectiveness. This expectation, which can affect performance, is called the _____ effect.

D. Ex Post Facto Designs

With ex post facto designs, the experimenter does not manipulate an independent variable but selects participants who naturally differ on some _____ variable. Ex post facto studies cannot demonstrate cause and effect.

III. Research Methods in Epidemiology

That branch of _____ that investigates factors contributing to the occurrence of a disease in a particular population is called epidemiology. When epidemiologists talk about the proportion of the population affected by a particular disease at a particular time, they use the term _____, and when they talk about the number of new cases of a disease during a particular time, they use the term _____.

A. Observational Methods

Research methods in epidemiology are similar to those used in psychology. Observational methods parallel _____ studies in psychology. The two types of observational methods are (1) studies that begin with a group of people already suffering from

16

a disease, and are called _____ studies, and (2) longitudinal studies that

follow the forward development of a group of people and are called

_____ studies. Some retrospective studies are called

_____-_____ studies because cases (people with a disease) are

compared to controls (people not affected).

B. Randomized, Controlled Trials

Randomized, controlled trials are equivalent to _____ in psychology.

These studies are often considered the "gold standard" of research design because they are

randomized, placebo-controlled, _____ - _____

designs that indicate cause and effect.

C. Natural Experiments

Natural experiments are similar to _____ studies in psychology—

both involve the selection rather than the manipulation of a variable. Natural experiments can

be conducted when two similar groups of people naturally divide themselves into those

exposed and those not exposed to a pathogen.

D. Meta-analysis

The statistical technique of _____-_____ allows researchers to

evaluate many research studies on the same topic, even if the research methods differed.

E. An Example of Epidemiological Research: The Alameda County Study

An example of epidemiological research is the Alameda County Study. Epidemiologists

have been studying the health effects of certain lifestyles of people in Alameda County (in

and around Oakland) for 40 years. They found that people who practiced six or seven basic

health-related behaviors were less likely to die than those who practiced zero to three. These

behaviors included (1) getting seven or eight hours of sleep daily, (2) eating breakfast almost

every day, (3) rarely eating between meals, (4) drinking alcohol in moderation or not at all,

(5) not _____, (6) exercising regularly, and (7) maintaining _____

near the prescribed ideal.

IV. Determining Causation

Most epidemiological studies do not demonstrate causation; rather, they point to specific

_____ factors that are associated with a particular disease or disorder.

A. The Risk Factor Approach

A risk factor is any characteristic or condition that occurs with greater frequency in people

with a disease than it does in people free from that disease. Although risk factors do not

determine causation, they can be used to estimate the _____ of people

developing a disease. Both relative risk and absolute risk are important.

_____ risk refers to a person's chance of developing a disease

independent of other people's chances. The ratio between the number of people in an exposed

group who have a disease and the number in an unexposed group with the disease is called

_____ risk.

B. Cigarettes and Disease: Is There a Causal Relationship?

Experimental designs give scientists their best method for determining

_____ ; that is, cause and effect. Although other research designs do not

independently determine causation, cumulative evidence from nonexperimental designs can

strongly suggest causal relationships, such as between smoking and developing disease. First,

the more people smoke, the more they are likely to suffer from a disease. This is called a

_____ -_____ relationship. Second, the prevalence and incidence of a

disease declines when people _____ smoking. Third, cigarette smoking

_____ development of disease rather than vice versa. Forth, the relationship

between cigarette smoking and disease makes sense from a _____ viewpoint.

Fifth, relevant research yields a consistent pattern of results—a pattern that has been

established through _____ -_____ , a statistical technique that allows the

combination of information from several studies into one analysis. Sixth, the size of the

relative risk is large—about 2.0 for cardiovascular disease and 23.0 for _____

_____ . Seventh, the evidence is based on a number of well-designed studies. A

18

combination of these criteria can allow epidemiologists to determine causality from nonexperimental designs.

V. Research Tools

Theories and psychometric methods are important tools for researchers.

A. The Role of Theory in Research

A set of related assumptions that allows scientists to use logical deductive reasoning to formulate testable hypotheses is one definition of a _____. Theories allow researchers to (1)_____ data, (2) render them meaningful, (3) generate descriptive research, (4) suggest a variety of _____ that can be tested, and (5) follow a guideline for working through daily problems.

B. The Role of Psychometrics in Research

Health psychologists, like other scientists, use measuring instruments to test their hypotheses and build their theories. To be useful, measuring devices must be both _____ (consistent) and _____ (accurate).

Multiple Choice Questions

_____ 1. An inactive substance or condition that can bring about positive change in people's performance is called a
   a. double-blind research design.
   b. a hypnotic suggestion.
   c. nocebo.
   d. placebo.

_____ 2. While listening to a morning television program, you hear a TV personality report that he lost 25 pounds as a result of self-hypnosis. Such a report
   a. is good evidence of the effectiveness of self-hypnosis in weight loss.
   b. should be considered a testimonial and given little or no credibility.
   c. should be considered as a case study.
   d. is an example of an ex post facto study.

19

_____ 3. Another term for placebo effect is _____ effect.
   a. nocebo
   b. double-blind
   c. randomized
   d. self-efficacy
   e. expectancy

_____ 4. The strength of the placebo effect is not always the same, but the average effect of a placebo is about _____ %.
   a. 10
   b. 29
   c. 35
   d. 50
   e. 75

_____ 5. When neither the participants in a study nor the experimenters know who is receiving the treatment and who is receiving a placebo, the experiment is a _____ design.
   a. double-blind
   b. randomized trial
   c. single-blind
   d. case study

_____ 6. As X increases, Y also increases; as X decreases, Y also decreases. Therefore, X and Y are
   a. negatively correlated.
   b. positively correlated.
   c. unrelated.
   d. none of the above.

_____ 7. A study that uses participants of at least two different age groups or developmental periods is called a(n)
   a. experimental study.
   b. ex post facto design.
   c. longitudinal study.
   d. cross-sectional study.

_____ 8. An important disadvantage of longitudinal studies is that they
   a. fail to take developmental trends into consideration.
   b. are time consuming.
   c. are limited to retrospective designs.
   d. are limited to ex post facto designs.

_____ 9. Which of these is the best example of a longitudinal study?
    a. a survey that compares the responses of college freshmen with those of their grandparents on attitudes toward health care
    b. a clinical trial that shows that AZT is an effective drug for slowing the rate of HIV infection
    c. a study that finds that level of education is inversely related to death rate from cardiovascular disease
    d. a study that follows the history of overweight in female participants over a 20-year period

_____ 10. An investigator measures blood pressure in a group of overweight 8th-grade students and overweight college seniors. This study is an example of
    a. a longitudinal study.
    b. a cross-sectional study.
    c. an experimental study.
    d. a clinical trial.

_____ 11. Researchers use _____ when their goal is to determine the cause of a disease.
    a. single-participant designs
    b. case-control studies
    c. correlational studies
    d. experimental designs

_____ 12. In a study that examines the effects of different types of exercise on body mass index, exercise would be
    a. the dependent variable.
    b. the independent variable.
    c. a placebo effect.
    d. an extraneous variable.

_____ 13. An experimental study examined the effects of weight loss on blood pressure in middle-aged men. The dependent variable in this study is
    a. gender.
    b. age.
    c. weight loss.
    d. blood pressure.

_____ 14. To determine if Drug X lowers blood pressure, scientists would administer Drug X to an experimental group and _____ to a comparison group.
    a. a placebo
    b. epinephrine
    c. a lower dose of Drug X
    d. a higher dose of Drug X

_____15. With regard to the placebo effect, one can most accurately say that it is
   a. physiologically real but not capable of alleviating organic symptoms.
   b. physiologically real and capable of alleviating organic as well as psychological symptoms.
   c. most likely to be manifested in well-designed experiments.
   d. an imaginary effect and thus not important.

_____16. Research designs that involve the selection of levels of a subject variable rather than the manipulation of levels of an independent variable are called
   a. ex post facto designs.
   b. correlational studies.
   c. cross-sectional studies.
   d. case studies.

_____17. The branch of medicine that investigates factors contributing to increased health or the occurrence of disease in a particular population is called
   a. health psychology.
   b. statistical health analysis.
   c. public health.
   d. epidemiology.

_____18. The number of new cases of AIDS in a given year is called
   a. rate of illness.
   b. rate of death.
   c. prevalence.
   d. incidence.

_____19. The percentage of the population that has a disease in any one period of time is called
   a. incidence.
   b. prevalence.
   c. correlational evidence.
   d. an epidemic.

_____20. Retrospective studies
   a. are a type of correlational study.
   b. begin with a group of participants who are disease-free and then follow them for a number of years.
   c. begin with a group of participants who already have a disease.
   d. are a type of case study.

_____21. Observational methods in epidemiology parallel _____ methods in psychology.
   a. correlational
   b. experimental
   c. cross-sectional
   d. case study
   e. none of the above

22

_____ 22. A prospective epidemiological study would also be
   a. longitudinal.
   b. correlational.
   c. cross-sectional.
   d. none of the above.

_____ 23. In a case-control study,
   a. people affected by a disease are compared with people not affected by that disease.
   b. one person is studied in detail over a short period of time.
   c. one person is studied on one characteristic over a long period of time.
   d. the responses of one group of people are correlated with the responses of another group.

_____ 24. Any condition that occurs with greater frequency in people with a disease than in people free from that disease is known as
   a. a correlational factor.
   b. a placebo effect.
   c. an extraneous variable.
   d. a risk factor.
   e. none of the above.

_____ 25. A woman who has a risk factor for cardiovascular disease
   a. will develop cardiovascular disease if she lives long enough.
   b. will not develop cardiovascular disease unless she has two or more risk factors.
   c. is more likely to develop cardiovascular disease than someone without the risk factor.
   d. exhibits some of the behavioral as well as some of the physical causes for cardiovascular disease.

_____ 26. When people are allowed to decide to be in either the experimental group or the control group, _____ becomes a serious problem.
   a. the placebo effect
   b. the ethical treatment of human participants
   c. the double-blind effect
   d. self-selection

_____ 27 Morbidity is to mortality as
   a. illness is to disease.
   b. disease is to death.
   c. death is to disease.
   d. death is to trauma.

_____28. You hear on the radio that researchers have found a significant negative correlation between eating tomatoes and developing prostate cancer. From this, you can conclude
   a. that eating tomatoes causes lower rates of prostate cancer.
   b. that eating tomatoes causes higher rates of prostate cancer.
   c. nothing about cause and effect.
   d. that the study was an experimental design.

_____29. Which studies best determine cause and effect?
   a. cross-sectional
   b. case studies
   c. experimental designs
   d. clinical trials

_____30. One function of a useful theory is to
   a. introduce bias in research.
   b. eliminate bias in research.
   c. generate research.
   d. be proven true.

_____31. The more cigarettes a man smokes, the greater his risk of heart disease. This description is an example of
   a. a dose-response relationship.
   b. a cause and effect relationship.
   c. an experimental study.
   d. a case-control study.
   e. a meta-analytical study.

_____32. To be valid, a test must be
   a. consistent.
   b. accurate.
   c. reliable.
   d. all of these.

Key Terms

Define each of the following:

correlational studies —

dependent variable —

dose-response relationship —

incidence —

independent variable —

placebo —

prevalence —

prospective study —

risk factor —

retrospective study —

Matching

Match the following:

1. Framingham study

    a. neither participants nor researchers know who received a placebo and who receives treatment

2. meta-analysis

    b. proportion of the population affected by a particular disease

3. seven behaviors related to health

    c. negative effects due to expectancy

4. double-blind technique

    d. Alameda County Study

5. ex post facto design

    e. independent and dependent variables

6. nocebo

    f. expressed as a correlation coefficient

7. prevalence

    g. demonstrated the importance of risk factors for heart disease

8. incidence

    h. subject variable

9. experimental designs

    i. statistical technique used to analyze a combination of many studies at once

10. test reliability

    j. number of new cases of a disease within a time period

1. _____ 2. _____ 3. _____ 4. _____ 5. _____

6. _____ 7. _____ 8. _____ 9. _____ 10. _____

Experimental Design—Can Counseling Help People Lower Their Fat Intake?

Your textbook includes an example of an experimental design that manipulates counseling as the independent variable and measures dietary fat as the dependent variable. Figure 2.1 shows this design which will allow researchers to answer the question, "Is counseling effective in helping people change their diet?"

In the figure that follows, fill in the missing information for an experiment to determine the influence of a low-fat diet on lowering cholesterol level. In this study, the type of diet (low-fat versus regular) is the independent variable, and change in cholesterol level is the dependent variable. Complete the missing information.

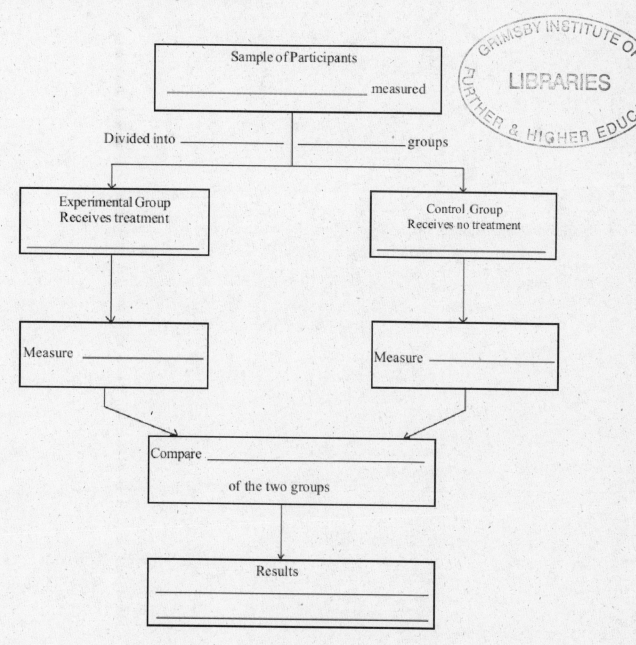

Essay Questions

1. What is a placebo, and how can it affect research and treatment?

2. Your friend Michelle learns that she has a risk factor for diabetes, and this news upsets her. What can you and Michelle conclude from the knowledge that she has a risk factor? What conclusions would be unwarranted?

Let's Get Personal—
Epidemiologists at Work

Your opportunities to be involved in epidemiology research are few, but you can see a dramatization of some very important epidemiology research by seeing *And the Band Played On*, which is available on DVD and video. This movie depicts the development of the AIDS epidemic and the search for its cause by the epidemiologists at the Centers for Disease Control and Prevention. In addition to the political complexities, the movie shows the field and laboratory research that identified the human immunodeficiency virus.

How did the CDC initially become aware that some new disease was spreading?

How did epidemiologists identify the modes of transmission for HIV infection?

How did epidemiologists identify the risk factors for HIV infection?

What were the barriers that slowed the identification of the modes of transmission and risk factors?

In addition to epidemiologists, what researchers were involved with understanding AIDS?

Answers

Fill in the Rest of the Story

I.   expectancy
I.A.   35; nocebo
I.B.   double-blind
II.A.   descriptive; -1.00; $+1.00$ (or $+1.00$; -1.00); cause
II.B.   ages; longitudinal; developmental
II.C.   independent; dependent; placebo
II.D.   subject (participant)
III.   medicine; prevalence; incidence
III.A.   descriptive; retrospective; prospective; case-control
III.B.   experimental; double-blind
III.C.   ex post facto
III.D.   meta-analysis
III.E.   smoking; weight
IV.   risk
IV.A.   probability (chance); Absolute; relative
IV.B.   causation; dose-response; quit (stop); precedes; biological; meta-analysis; lung cancer
V.A.   theory; organize; hypotheses
V.B.   reliable; valid

Multiple Choice

1.	d	9.	d	17.	d	25.	c
2.	b	10.	b	18.	d	26.	d
3.	e	11.	d	19.	b	27.	b
4.	c	12.	b	20.	c	28.	c
5.	a	13.	d	21.	a	29.	c
6.	b	14.	a	22.	a	30.	c
7.	d	15.	b	23.	a	31.	a
8.	b	16.	a	24.	d	32.	d

Matching

1.	g	2.	i	3.	d	4.	a	5.	h
6.	c	7.	b	8.	j	9.	e	10.	f

Good points to include in your essay answers:

1. A placebo is a treatment that is capable of causing effects through expectation of the effectiveness of the treatment, independent of the influence of the treatment itself. It has effects for both research and treatment.
   A. Placebo effects in research present problems.
      1. People expect treatments to work and respond according to their expectancies rather than according to the treatment.
      2. The response to placebos creates an inflated assessment of the effectiveness of both medical and psychological treatment.
      3. Researchers must include some control procedures to allow for the accurate assessment of treatment effectiveness, usually a "blind" procedure.
   B. Placebo effects are an advantage in treatment situations.
      1. Placebos bring about improvements and cures that are indistinguishable from those brought about by medically and psychologically effective treatments.
      2. The placebo effect can add to the effect of medical and psychological treatment, boosting the effectiveness.

2. A risk factor is some characteristic or condition that occurs with greater frequency in people with a disease than in people without the disease.
   A. Knowing that Michelle has a risk factor allows you to conclude that
      1. Her risk for developing diabetes is elevated.
      2. She is more likely to develop diabetes than someone without the risk factor.
   B. Knowing that Michelle has a risk factor does not reveal that
      1. She is certain to develop diabetes.
      2. This or any other risk factor is the cause of diabetes.

CHAPTER 3
Seeking Health Care

Learning Objectives

After studying Chapter 3, you should be able to

1. Evaluate the models that attempt to explain health-related behaviors.

2. Distinguish between illness behavior and sick role behavior.

3. Discuss the cognitive and demographic factors that affect seeking health care.

4. Identify the factors that people consider when choosing a health care practitioner.

5. Describe the problems that people encounter when receiving medical care.

Fill in the Rest of the Story

I. Adopting Health-Related Behaviors

Although health is highly valued, people do not always behave in ways that promote their health.

A. Theories of Health-Protective Behaviors

Several theories attempt to explain health-related behaviors. The health belief model includes four factors that should combine to predict health-related behaviors: perceived susceptibility to disease or disability, perceived severity of the disease or disability, perceived _____ of health-enhancing behaviors, and perceived _____ to health-enhancing behaviors.

The theory of reasoned action assumes that people are quite reasonable and make systematic use of information when deciding how to behave. According to this theory, the immediate determinant of behavior is a person's _____ to act, which in turn is shaped by one's attitude toward the behavior and one's perception of the social pressure to perform or not perform the action; that is, one's _____.

The theory of planned behavior is an extension of the theory of reasoned action, adding people's perception of their control over behavior. The ease or difficulty of achieving desired behavioral outcomes is called perceived _____ control and reflects both past behaviors and perceived ability to overcome obstacles.

Neil Weinstein's _____ adoption process model assumes that when people begin new and relatively complex behaviors aimed at protecting themselves from harm, they go through as many as seven stages of belief about their personal susceptibility. In Stage 1, people are unaware of the hazard. In Stage 2, they are aware of the hazard but believe that, although others are at risk, they are not at risk—a situation Weinstein calls an _____ _____. People in Stage 3 acknowledge their _____ and accept the notion that precaution would be personally effective. Action occurs in Stage 4, whereas in the parallel Stage 5, people decide that action is _____. In Stage 6, people have already taken the precaution aimed at reducing risks, and Stage 7 involves _____ the precaution.

B. Critique of Health-Related Theories

How do these health-related theories meet criteria of a useful theory; that is, how well do they (1) generate _____, (2) organize and _____ observations, and (3) help the practitioner predict and change behaviors? None of the models are able to completely explain the complexities of health-related behavior.

II. Seeking Medical Attention

How people determine their health status when they don't feel well depends on their social and cultural background, their interpretation of symptoms, and their concept of what constitutes illness. Those activities, by people who feel sick, that are directed toward determining health status before an official diagnosis are called _____ behaviors, whereas those activities exhibited by people after they have been diagnosed that are aimed at trying to get well are _____ _____ behaviors.

34

A. Illness Behavior

Many people have a personal reluctance to seek medical care. They are willing to advise others to see a doctor, but with the same symptoms, they are _____ to go to the doctor themselves. Several social and demographic factors predict willingness to seek professional care. One is gender; _____ are more likely than _____ to seek health care. Socioeconomic level is another factor; people with higher incomes are less likely than those with lower incomes to become sick, but they are _____ likely to seek health care and to do so more quickly when they become ill. Young and middle-aged people show more reluctance to seek health care than older adults. Stress is also a factor in seeking health care, and stress _____ the likelihood of seeking health care.

Symptom characteristics also influence how people respond to illness. People are most likely to seek medical care when their symptoms are visible to themselves and to others, when they view the symptoms as _____, when their symptoms interfere with their usual _____, and when their symptoms recur or _____.

Howard Leventhal and his colleagues identified five components in the conceptualization of illness. First is the identity of the disease. People need to label their symptoms, and such a label seems to _____ anxieties. Second, the _____ _____ helps people conceptualize illness. When people receive a diagnosis, they think about the time course of both the disease and the treatment. Third, people attribute a _____ to their symptoms. Fourth, they think of the consequences of their disease, and fifth, they consider the controllability of their illness.

B. The Sick Role

After people become convinced that they are ill, they adopt the _____ _____. Sick people are usually exempt from attending school, going to

35

work, cooking meals, or cleaning house. Their obligations include acting

_____ while also using health care services to get better.

III. Receiving Health Care

The expense of health care has led to restricted access for most U.S. residents. Those

people who have health _____ receive better care and have more choices about their

health care than people who do not. However, the rise of managed care and the increasing health

care costs have made health care less accessible.

A. Limited Access to Health Care

In 1965, the U.S. Congress created two programs to provide health care; the first is

Medicare, which pays hospital expenses for most Americans over the age of

_____. The second program was _____, which provides health

care based on low income and physical problems.

B. Choosing a Practitioner

Part of seeking health care is choosing a practitioner—a physician or one of the many

alternative types of health care practitioners. As medicine has become more complex,

technological, and corporate, patients have adopted a _____ attitude

toward medicine. For many poor people, their only experience of receiving health care is

going to a hospital _____ room where they receive care when they are

sicker than they might have been if they had easier access to care.

C. The Rise of Managed Health Care

HMOs, or _____ _____ _____ were organized to

provide affordable care by keeping people healthy. However, they evolved into

organizations in which staff physicians are gatekeepers, which makes it more difficult for

patients to see a medical specialist. Insurance companies have also played a role in

managed care. Many insurance plans now have lists of preferred or exclusive providers

whom members may consult. If members wish to choose a practitioner not on the list, they

will have a greater _____ burden.

D. Being in the Hospital

Being in the hospital can be a stressful experience for several reasons. In addition to being sick, hospitalized patients must cope with the hospital routine and deal with the possibility of distressing medical procedures. Being a patient means conforming to rules of the health care institution and complying with medical advice. Many hospitalized patients become almost invisible to the hospital staff and are treated as though they were not present; that is, they receive _____ treatment. Well-informed patients tend to be less stressed than poorly informed ones, but traditionally hospitalized patients have experienced a _____ of information about their condition. Patients who must conform to hospital routine and are not allowed to make everyday decisions experience a loss of _____, which often adds more stress to an already stressful situation.

Children are especially vulnerable to persistent fears as a result of receiving medical treatment. Familiarization with procedures, modeling, and cognitive behavioral techniques can decrease children's fears. However, these interventions add to _____, which limits their use.

Multiple Choice Questions

_____ 1. Psychologists use theories to
    a. predict behavior.
    b. explain behavior.
    c. both a and b.
    d. neither a nor b.

_____ 2. The theory that includes the concepts of perceived susceptibility to disease, perceived severity of the disease, perceived benefits of health-enhancing behaviors, and perceived barriers to health-enhancing behaviors is
    a. the theory of planned behavior.
    b. the theory of reasoned action.
    c. the precaution adoption process model.
    d. the health belief model.

37

_____ 3. The _____ assumes that the immediate cause of people's actions is their intention to act.
   a. health belief model
   b. transtheoretical model
   c. precaution adoption process model
   d. theory of reasoned action

_____ 4. According to the theory of reasoned action, a person's perception of the social pressure to perform or not perform an action is called
   a. perceived severity of one's illness.
   b. subjective norm.
   c. attitude toward the behavior.
   d. optimistic bias.

_____ 5. Which of these concepts is crucial to the theory of reasoned action?
   a. internal locus of control
   b. perceived severity of the disease
   c. intention to act
   d. perceived susceptibility to a disease

_____ 6. Perceived behavioral control is a key concept in the
   a. transtheoretical model.
   b. behavior modification approach.
   c. theory of reasoned action.
   d. theory of planned behavior.

_____ 7. Neil Weinstein suggested that, when people begin new and relatively complex behaviors aimed at protecting themselves from harm, they go through a series of beliefs about their personal susceptibility. This model of behavior is called the
   a. the transtheoretical model.
   b. theory of planned behavior.
   c. self-regulation theory.
   d. the precaution adoption process model.

_____ 8. Austin, like most of his friends, does not exercise regularly. He believes that his sedentary friends are susceptible to heart disease, but he exempts himself from any high risk. Weinstein would say that Austin
   a. will take action to protect himself.
   b. is in Stage 6 of the adoption precaution process.
   c. has an optimistic bias.
   d. will eventually develop heart disease.

_____ 9. Models of health-protective behavior have limitations in predicting health-seeking behavior, but
    a. the health belief model is superior to the other models.
    b. these models predict better than chance.
    c. psychologists have not been involved in the development of these models.
    d. theory of reasoned action generated little research.

_____ 10. Older models of health-seeking behaviors have generally not performed well in predicting behavior. One reason for this situation is that the theories often do not take _____ into consideration.
    a. severity of the illness
    b. cultural factors such as racism and poverty
    c. internal locus of control
    d. social norms
    e. optimistic bias

_____ 11. After feeling ill for two days, Angelo went to his doctor who diagnosed his illness as influenza and prescribed bed rest and medication. Angelo had the prescription filled, took the medication, and went to bed. Angelo's behavior after seeing his doctor would be considered
    a. illness behavior.
    b. sick role behavior.
    c. reluctance behavior.
    d. reactance behavior.

_____ 12. People's actions designed to determine their health status are called
    a. sick role behaviors.
    b. illness behaviors.
    c. health-seeking behaviors.
    d. premature diagnoses.

_____ 13. Which of these persons is MOST likely to seek health care?
    a. a 14-year-old boy with a bruise on his shoulder
    b. a 6-year-old girl with a temperature of 100.5°
    c. a middle-aged man with a sore knee
    d. a 48-year old woman who suffers from asthma attacks

_____ 14. People in high socioeconomic levels are _____ likely than other people to have symptoms and _____ likely to go to health care professionals when they do.
    a. more . . . less
    b. more . . . more
    c. less . . . more
    d. less . . . less

_____15. Research on seeking health care suggests that if both Kyle and Cameron are experiencing similar discomfort but Kyle has visible symptoms, then
   a. Kyle is more likely than Cameron to seek health care.
   b. both Kyle and Cameron will make an appointment with a physician.
   c. Cameron is likely to seek health care, but Kyle is not.
   d. Kyle is likely to seek alternative health care, and Cameron is likely to see a physician.

_____16. Howard Leventhal and his associates consider _____ to be a component in people's conceptualization of illness.
   a. the monetary cost of treatment
   b. the consequence of the illness
   c. the competence level of the physician
   d. all of the above

_____17. Dustin has not been feeling well lately. In trying to diagnose himself, Dustin is likely to
   a. deny the existence of his symptoms.
   b. try to find a nonthreatening label that fits his symptoms.
   c. exaggerate his symptoms so as to imagine the most serious consequences.
   d. repress his symptoms.

_____18. Which of these programs was designed to help people over the age of 65 afford health care?
   a. Medicare
   b. Medicaid
   c. Metropolitan Life Insurance
   c. the Socialized Medicine Act of 1997

_____19. Patients who choose female physicians may expect
   a. to receive lower quality care than those who choose male physicians.
   b. to be kept waiting longer in the waiting room than those who choose male physicians.
   c to spend more time with their physicians than those who choose male physicians.
   d. a similar level of impersonal treatment from male and female physicians.

_____20. Poor people in need of health care are likely to receive such care
   a. in an emergency room.
   b. from a psychologist.
   c. from an osteopath.
   d. from a chiropractor.

_____21. The original rationale behind health maintenance organizations (HMOs) was that
   a. every American should have health insurance.
   b. prevention of an illness is preferable to treatment of the illness.
   c. more physicians should be women.
   d. every American over the age of 65 should have free health care.

_____ 22. Health maintenance organizations have had several important impacts on health care in the United States. Which of these is NOT a result of the growth of HMOs?
   a. People have greater choice in selecting their health care providers.
   b. The authority of physicians has been diminished.
   c. More physicians practice with a team of health care providers.
   d. Physicians have less choice in managing their patients' health care.

_____ 23. Which of the following has led to a DECREASE in patient satisfaction?
   a. a decrease in the number of HMOs and an increase in the number of private physicians
   b. an increase in the availability of alternative medicine providers and a increase in insurance coverage for these services
   c. an increase in the Medicare payments combined with an increased number of people insured by private companies
   d. the growth of managed care and the restriction of access to health services

_____ 24. During the past 25 years,
   a. the number of surgeries and tests performed on an outpatient basis has dropped dramatically.
   b. technology to diagnose illnesses has become much more sophisticated.
   c. hospital stays have become longer.
   d. patients have become more restrained in voicing their concerns to their physicians.

_____ 25. From the point of view of the hospital staff, the ideal patient would be
   a. very intelligent.
   b. very talkative.
   c. unconscious.
   d. dead.
   e. robot-like.

_____ 26. In the United States, the number of deaths each year from medical errors has been estimated to be from about
   a. 10,000 to 12,000.
   b. 20,000 to 30,000.
   c. 30,000 to 40,000.
   d. 44,000 to 98,000.

_____ 27. Even when prescribed and taken properly, prescription drugs account for between _____ and _____ deaths each year in the United States.
   a. 5,000 . . . 7,000
   b. 13,000 . . . 18,000
   c. 22,000. . . 27,000
   d. 47,000 . . . 56,000
   e. 76,000 . . . 137,000

_____28. Tomorrow morning Candice's daughter Laura is scheduled for surgery to remove a benign tumor. Because Laura is anxious about the surgery, Candice reassures her by saying, "Everything will turn out fine. You have nothing to worry about. It won't hurt." These words are likely to
   a. increase Laura's fear and anxiety.
   b. decrease Laura's anxiety but increase her fear.
   c. decrease Laura's fear and anxiety.
   d. allow Laura to sleep well tonight.

Key Terms

Define each of the following:

illness behavior —

Health belief model —

Theory of reasoned action —

Theory of planned behavior —

Precaution adoption process model —

sick role behavior —

Medicare —

Medicaid —

HMO —

nonperson treatment —

Matching

Match the following:

1. optimistic bias

2. illness behavior

3. sick role behavior

4. health belief model

5. theory of reasoned action

6. extension of theory of reasoned action

7. components of illness conceptualization

8. Medicare

9. Medicaid

a. components include attitudes, intentions, and subjective norms

b. behavior after receiving a diagnosis

c. components include susceptibility, severity, perceived benefits, and perceived barriers

d. provides health care to those with low income

e. pays hospital expenses for people over 65

f. precaution adoption process model

g. activities undertaken to determine health status

h. visibility of symptoms and perceived severity of symptoms

i. theory of planned behavior

1. _____ 2. _____ 3. _____ 4. _____ 5. _____

6. _____ 7. _____ 8. _____ 9. _____

Theory of Reasoned Action in Action

Austin has been thinking about beginning an exercise program to attain a higher level of physical fitness. He has always thought that running or jogging is the best exercise, but his friend Tyler tells him that weightlifting is an excellent exercise. Not only does weight training lead to better fitness, but it also helps in building upper body strength and improves appearance. Austin considers the advantages of weightlifting and concludes that he would like that type of exercise better than jogging. He wonders about the availability of weightlifting equipment and visits the college gym to examine their equipment. The next time he sees Tyler, Austin tells him that he is considering weight training, and Tyler invites Austin to come to the gym with him the next day. Austin agrees, and they meet at the gym the next day.

Fill in each of the boxes in the figure to match Austin's adoption of an exercise program to the theory of reasoned action:

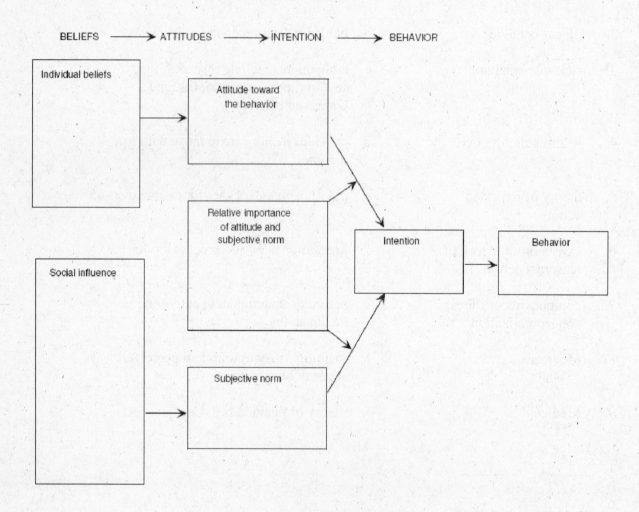

Essay Questions

1. What role do the theories of health-protective behavior serve? How successful are these theories?

2. How has the rise of managed health care changed the health care that people receive?

Let's Get Personal— What Is Sick?

Your personal view of illness affects your behavior when you believe that you are ill. That personal view depends on your knowledge about various diseases and your cognitions about illness. As various researchers have discovered, people who have a sophisticated knowledge about illness may still hold some irrational cognitions about illness.

To explore your illness beliefs, write a description of the last time you were sick. Choose an illness episode that was sufficiently severe to affect your daily routine and cause you to label yourself as sick.

Answer the following questions:

When was the last time you were sick?

What caused you to be sick?

What led you initially to believe that you were sick?

What were the symptoms you noticed?

Was there a time period in which you were not sure that you were sick? If so, what convinced you that you were ill?

Did you receive a diagnosis from a health care professional, or did you diagnose yourself?

How long were you sick?

What changes did you make in your daily activities because you were sick?

What was involved in getting well?

Did you exhibit the typical reluctance to seek medical care by avoiding contact with the medical profession, or did you go to the doctor when you initially experienced symptoms? In either case, what beliefs account for your behavior?

Research indicates that people label their symptoms so that they understand the identity of their illness and that this label is important in understanding the time course and severity of their illness. Is this research consistent with your experience?

When you described what caused you to be sick, did that explanation include a high level of biomedical knowledge? Research indicates that even students with a high level of biological knowledge tend to omit such detail and rely on behavioral factors to explain their illnesses. Is this research consistent with your experience?

Answers

Fill in the Rest of the Story

I.A.   benefits; barriers; intention; subjective norms; behavioral; precaution; optimistic bias; risk; unnecessary; maintaining

I.B.   research; explain

II.   illness; sick role

II.A.   reluctant (unwilling); women; men; more; increases; severe (serious); activities; persist; diminish (reduce, decrease); time line; cause

II.B.   sick role; sick

III.   insurance

III.A.   65; Medicaid

III.B.   consumer; emergency

III.C.   Health Maintenance Organizations; financial

III.D.   nonperson; lack; control; costs

Multiple Choice

1.	c	8.	c	15.	a	22.	a
2.	d	9.	b	16.	b	23.	d
3.	d	10.	b	17.	b	24.	b
4.	b	11.	b	18.	a	25.	e
5.	c	12.	b	19.	c	26.	d
6.	d	13.	d	20.	a	27.	e
7.	d	14.	c	21.	b	28.	a

Matching

1. f   2. g   3. b   4. c   5. a   6. i   7. h   8. e   9. d

Good points to include in your essay answers:

1.   A.   Like all theories, these should
       1.   Generate research.
       2.   Organize and explain behavior.
       3.   Help practitioners change behavior.
   B.   The health belief model, theory of reasoned action, theory of planned behavior, and the precaution adoption model have been only modestly successful in predicting health-related behaviors.
       1.   The health belief model and theory of reasoned action have generated quite a bit of research, but the support for these models has been no better than modest.
       2.   All these theories organize and explain behavior, but research has confirmed only some components of the models.

3. The theories are better at predicting health-seeking behavior than are demographic factors, but all of them leave a great deal unexplained.
4. With only partial support for any model and failure to explain many facets of health-seeking behavior, practical advice is difficult to formulate.

2. A. The rise of managed health care has restricted access to health care.
   1. HMOs have become major providers of health care, and these organizations limit access to services.
   2. People without insurance coverage have limited access to health care; people with insurance may be restricted to providers from a preferred list.
   B. The rise of managed care has affected interactions between health care providers and patients.
   1. Many physicians work in group practices or for HMOs, which emphasize cost containment.
   2. Practitioners spend less time with patients.
   3. Patients may not see the same practitioner on each health care visit, preventing the development of a relationship.
   C. Cost cutting measures have affected the experience of hospitalization.
   1. Outpatient treatment has increased, and hospital stays are shorter.
   2. Fewer staff care for more patients, increasing depersonalized treatment in the hospital setting.

CHAPTER 4
Adhering to Medical Advice

Learning Objectives

After studying Chapter 4, you should be able to

1. Evaluate the models that have been used to explain adherence.
2. Define adherence and provide information about how often people fail to adhere to medical advice.
3. Explain methods of measuring adherence.
4. Discuss what factors predict and fail to predict adherence.
5. Identify effective and ineffective strategies to improve adherence.

Fill in the Rest of the Story

I.   Theories That Apply to Adherence

Several theoretical models that apply to behavior in general have also been applied to the problem of adherence and nonadherence, including the behavioral model and several

_____ learning theories.

A. Behavioral Model

The behavioral model is based on the assumption that reinforcers strengthen behavior, whereas _____ inhibits or suppresses behavior. Advocates of the behavioral model use cues, _____, and contracts to reinforce compliant behaviors.

B. Self-Efficacy Theory

Albert Bandura's social cognitive theory emphasizes the interaction of environment, behavior, and person factors to predict human functioning. He calls this interaction _____ determinism. An important part of the person factor is one's perceived ability to perform behaviors necessary to bring about a desired consequence, a component Bandura calls _____-_____. Bandura emphasizes people's interpretation and evaluation of their situation, their emotional response, and their perceived ability to _____ with illness symptoms in a specific situation.

C. Theories of Reasoned Action and Planned Behavior

The theory of reasoned action and the theory of planned behavior both assume that _____ are the immediate determinants of behavior. The theory of reasoned action assumes that intentions are influenced by _____ toward the behavior, _____ norms, and the motivation to comply with these norms. The theory of planned behavior includes an additional determinant of intentions to act, namely, people's perception of how much _____ they have over their behavior. Both theories have been used to predict adherence to a number of health-related behaviors.

D. The Transtheoretical Model

The transtheoretical model of James Prochaska and his colleagues assumes that people progress through five stages in making changes in behavior: _____, contemplation, preparation, action, and _____. In the first stage, people may fail to see that they have a problem. People in the second stage are aware of the problem, have thought about changing their behavior, but have not yet taken action. During the _____ stage, people make specific plans to change behavior, but people in this stage have not yet made an effort to change. Modification of behavior comes in the _____ stage when people make overt changes in their behavior. During the _____ stage, people try to sustain the changes they have made and to resist temptation to relapse.

II. Issues in Adherence

Issues in adherence include definition, assessment, and frequency. Research indicates that people who fail to _____ to their medication regimens have poorer medical outcomes.

A. What Is Adherence?

Because the term *compliance* suggests reluctant obedience, many psychologists prefer *adherence,* but a more ideal term would be _____ or collaboration.

B. How Is Adherence Measured?

At least six methods have been used to assess patient compliance: (1) ask the clinician, (2) ask the _____, (3) ask other people, (4) count pills, (5) examine biochemical evidence, or combine two or more of these methods. All approaches have limitations, but the *least* valid method is to ask the _____ about rate of patient compliance.

C. How Frequent Is Nonadherence?

In general terms, the rate of nonadherence to medical or health advice is about _____ %. The rate of adherence _____ for some conditions such as HIV and arthritis treatments and _____ for some conditions such as diabetes.

III. What Factors Predict Adherence?

Several illness characteristics relate to compliance, but not necessarily the factors that seem obvious.

A. Severity of the Disease

_____ of the disease is not a reliable predictor of how well patients adhere to medical advice, but the person's *perception* of severity is more closely related to adherence. In addition, when patients experience _____, they are more likely to comply with medical recommendations.

B. Treatment Characteristics

Noncompliance tends to increase as duration of therapy _____. In general, the greater the variety of medications a person must take, the _____ the likelihood of nonadherence.

C. Personal Factors

Personal factors such as age, gender, personality patterns, emotional factors, and personal beliefs all relate to adherence. Age has a complex relationship with adherence, but older people have many _____ to adherence because of complex medication schedules. Few overall differences exist in compliance rates for women and men, but _____ are more likely to adhere to a healthy diet. Of the various personality variables investigated, no _____ personality trait has emerged as a predictor of adherence. Anxiety and _____ life events are also related to adherence—both _____ the rate of adherence, but _____ is even more strongly related to failures in compliance. Personal beliefs are also related to compliance. People who believe that they are personally responsible for their own health are _____ likely to adhere.

D. Environmental Factors

Environmental factors are a more important influence on adherence than personal factors are. Socioeconomic factors, including _____, affect the ability to pay for follow-up care and prescribed medications. Social support is one of the strongest predictors of adherence, and those with a _____ tend to adhere better than those with fewer relationships.

E. Cultural Norms

Cultural beliefs and attitudes are related to compliance. Patients whose beliefs are not consistent with Western medicine are less likely to follow the advice of _____. Also, cultural factors may influence the treatment patients receive. Hispanic American and African American patients who feel discriminated against are _____ likely to follow the advice of a provider they believe to be biased or disrespectful.

F. The Practitioner-Patient Interaction

Perhaps the best predictor of patient compliance is the quality of the _____ between practitioner and patient. When patients fail to receive information they have requested, their adherence _____. Patients may fail to remember or may misunderstand what their practitioners tell them, and communication difficulties are more likely to occur when patients and practitioners differ in language, _____, ethnic background, or social class.

Patients' compliance improves as confidence in their physician's _____ ability increases. Both male and female physicians improve adherence when they are friendly and willing to listen to the patient; _____ physicians are more likely to show these qualities.

G. Interaction of Factors

Many factors show a relationship to adherence, but the contribution of each is _____. Studying the mutual influences of factors and their _____ may lead to a fuller understanding of the factors that predict adherence.

IV. Improving Adherence

Adherence to medical advice is far from ideal, and improving adherence is an urgent priority.

A. What Are the Barriers to Adherence?

Many barriers prevent people from adhering to medical advice. Many people fail to follow their doctor's advice because they do not correctly hear or _____ that advice, they find the regimen too complex or difficult, or they stop taking medication when symptoms _____. Many patients have an _____ bias and believe that they will be spared the serious consequences of nonadherence. Using a broad definition, adherence demands difficult _____ changes, such as changing one's diet, quitting smoking, or beginning an exercise program, which are difficult to follow.

B. How Can Adherence Be Improved?

Procedures that impart information boost knowledge but do not usually result in increased compliance are called _____ strategies. Behavioral strategies have generally been found to be _____ effective than educational procedures in enhancing patient adherence. _____ interviewing is one such approach. Procedures that increase patient adherence include clearly _____ instructions, _____ to help people remember medication or appointments, regimens tailored to patient's daily schedule, rewards for compliant behavior, and providing a written _____ that specifies the responsibilities of both provider and patient.

Multiple Choice Questions

_____ 1. The behavioral model of adherence
a. includes the concept of subjective norms.
b. is less effective than support groups in reducing friction in families with adolescent diabetics.
c. emphasizes punishment of noncompliant behaviors.
d. emphasizes reinforcement of compliant behaviors.

_____ 2. Which of these reinforcers strengthens behavior?
a. positive
b. negative
c. punitive
d. both a and b
e. all of the above

_____ 3. A key element in Albert Bandura's model of reciprocal determinism is
a. subjective norms.
b. intention to behave.
c. self-efficacy.
d. internal locus of control.

_____ 4. According to Albert Bandura's idea of reciprocal determinism, human conduct is influenced by
a. behavior.
b. environment.
c. person factors.
d. an interaction among a, b, and c.

_____ 5. In the theory of reasoned action, behavioral intentions are a function of people's
   a. prior behavior.
   b. subjective norms.
   c. attitudes toward the behavior plus their subjective norms.
   d. optimistic bias.

_____ 6. When applied to compliance, _____ emphasizes rewards for compliant behaviors.
   a. the theory of reasoned action
   b. the behavioral model
   c. the adoption precaution process model
   d. the transtheoretical model

_____ 7. Celeste is 85 pounds overweight and has high blood pressure. She has never thought
   that her weight and blood pressure might be dangerous. According to the
   transtheoretical model, Celeste is at the _____ stage.
   a. final
   b. optimistic bias
   c. precontemplation
   d. maintenance

_____ 8. Tina is 25 pounds underweight, seldom eats more than three or four green beans a
   day, but she believes that she is too fat. According to Prochaska's transtheoretical
   model, the immediate strategy in this case should be designed to move Tina from the
   _____ stage to the _____ stage
   a. precontemplation . . . contemplation
   b. action . . . precontemplation
   c. maintenance . . . preparation
   d. contemplation . . . action

_____ 9. Larry smokes two packs of cigarettes a day. In recent weeks, he has thought seriously
   about quitting smoking. According to Prochaska's theory, Larry is at the _____ stage.
   a. contemplation
   b. action
   c. precontemplation
   d. self-efficacy

_____ 10. According to the transtheoretical model, the relapse process takes what shape?
   a. box
   b. triangle
   c. round
   d. spiral
   e. cone

_____ 11. Health psychologists often avoid the term *compliance* because it seems to suggest
    a. cooperation.
    b. defiance.
    c. yielding to outside pressure.
    d. withstanding harsh conditions.

_____ 12. Health psychologists suggest that the ideal relationship between patient and physician should be one of
    a. cooperation.
    b. compliance.
    c. obedience.
    d. reactance.

_____ 13. According to the broad definition of compliance discussed in your textbook, the following behavior would be regarded as compliant:
    a. smoking cigarettes.
    b. continuing to take medication as prescribed even after one's symptoms have disappeared.
    c. discontinuing medication when the symptoms disappear.
    d. failing to keep an appointment with an oncologist for fear of being diagnosed with cancer.

_____ 14. Research suggests that physicians tend to
    a. accurately estimate rate of patient compliance.
    b. underestimate rate of patient compliance.
    c. overestimate rate of patient compliance.
    d. be disinterested in rate of patient compliance.

_____ 15. A major difficulty of counting pills to measure compliance is that
    a. someone may not count unused pills accurately.
    b. the method is less reliable than physician judgment.
    c. the missing pills may not have been taken according to directions.
    d. seriously ill patients may not be motivated to count pills.

_____ 16. An advantage of examining biochemical evidence as a measure of adherence is that such evidence provides
    a. a reliable estimate of adherence.
    b. a valid estimate of adherence.
    c. a procedure that focuses on outcome.
    d. an inexpensive means of assessing adherence.

_____ 17. In general terms, methods of assessing patient compliance
    a. are quite reliable.
    b. are quite valid.
    c. are both reliable and valid.
    d. have problems with reliability and validity.

_____ 18. Rates of noncompliance differ according to a variety of factors, but generally these rates are about _____ %.
   a. 25
   b. 50
   c. 75
   d. 90

_____ 19. In general, higher rates for compliance occur when
   a. the medication is inexpensive.
   b. the medication is for prevention.
   c. the medication is for curing a disease.
   d. patients have no visible symptoms.

_____ 20. Kevin takes the medication prescribed for his condition only infrequently. Kevin's condition probably
   a. has not yet been diagnosed.
   b. is not very painful.
   c. is not a chronic disease.
   d. is not a hereditary disorder.

_____ 21. With regard to noncompliance, which of these statements most clearly agrees with research findings?
   a. Unpleasant side effects of an HIV drug therapy are unrelated to dropping out of a treatment regimen.
   b. The more complex a treatment regimen, the greater the likelihood that people will fail to comply.
   c. People suffering from a chronic illness are more likely to be compliant than those suffering from an acute illness.
   d. People with no visible symptoms are more likely to be compliant than people with obvious symptoms.

_____ 22. With regard to personal characteristics, research suggests that
   a. people past 80 have high rates of compliance to cancer screening.
   b. women and men show similar rates of compliance.
   c. younger people have more barriers to compliance than older individuals.
   d. people with a large network of friends are less likely than other people to adhere to medical advice.

_____ 23. Research on the link between personality traits and compliance rates has shown
   a. no evidence of a noncompliant personality.
   b. that people who are depressed are more compliant than people who are not.
   c. personality pattern is more important than the situation in predicting compliance.
   d. that women have noncompliant personalities, but men do not.

_____ 24. Which of these conditions is related to high rates of adherence?
   a. high levels of anxiety
   b. a high number of stressful life events
   c. a strong belief in the efficacy of the treatment
   d. having an authoritarian male physician

_____ 25. Which of the following approaches is generally LEAST effective in improving compliance rates?
   a. educational messages.
   b. cues.
   c. rewards.
   d. tailoring the regimen to the patient's daily routine.

_____ 26. Which of the following approaches is generally MOST effective in improving compliance rates?
   a. verbal punishments
   b. educational messages
   c. simple, clearly written instructions
   d. rational explanations concerning the dire consequences of noncompliance

_____ 27. Email reminders to take medication are classified as
   a. educational strategies to boost compliance.
   b. motivational interviewing.
   c. a combination of educational and placebo training.
   d. a behavioral strategy that uses prompts to boost compliance.

Key Terms

Define each of the following:

adherence —

behavioral model of compliance —

compliance —

motivational interviewing —

negative reinforcement —

positive reinforcement —

punishment —

self-efficacy theory —

transtheoretical model —

Matching

Match the following:

1. self-efficacy

2. includes an intentions component

3. precontemplation and maintenance

4. includes a control component

5. positive and negative reinforcement

6. the behavioral model

7. prompts and contingency contracts

8. poor predictor of adherence

9. good predictor of adherence

a. strengthen behavior, including compliance

b. improve compliance

c. severity of the disease

d. the theory of reasoned action and the theory of planned behavior

e. painful symptoms

f. proposes that reinforcement and punishment affect compliance

g. the transtheoretical model

h. the theory of planned behavior

i. specific to the situation rather than a global trait

1. _____ 2. _____ 3. _____ 4. _____ 5. _____

6. _____ 7. _____ 8. _____ 9. _____

Understanding the Transtheoretical Model

To better understand the transtheoretical model, apply it to the process of adopting a low-calorie diet by labeling the stages that correspond to each statement.

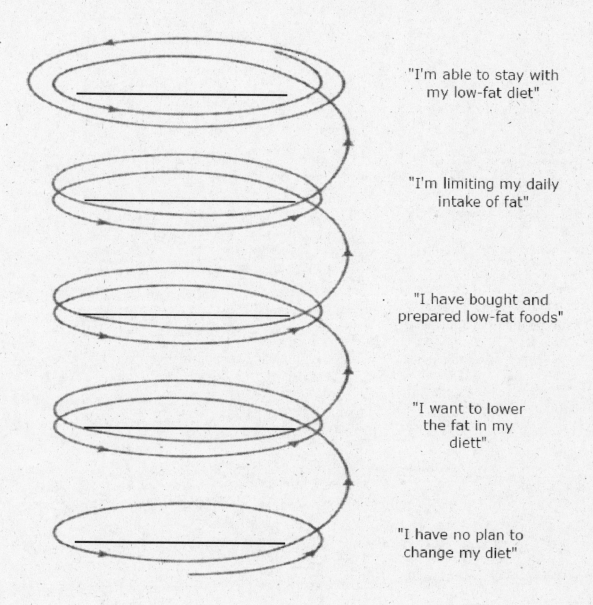

"I'm able to stay with my low-fat diet"

"I'm limiting my daily intake of fat"

"I have bought and prepared low-fat foods"

"I want to lower the fat in my diett"

"I have no plan to change my diet"

Essay Questions

1. Marissa is a college student who began an aerobics exercise program three weeks ago. Analyze her behavior using the transtheoretical model.

2. Which is more important in compliance—the person's personality or the person's social circumstances?

Let's Get Personal—
What's Your Problem with Compliance?

Unless you are exceptional, you fail to comply with some aspect of exemplary health behavior. Perhaps you have a medicine cabinet full of bottles with only a few pills, indicating that you have failed to take your medication as prescribed. Perhaps you have not had a physical examination in years. Perhaps you eat a high-fat diet, smoke, or fail to exercise regularly. Almost everyone deviates from medical orders in some respect.

Sometimes the problem is knowledge and the failure to understand what is required to follow medical advice. More often, some situational barriers prevent people from doing what they know they should do. Choose a noncompliant behavior and analyze the barriers that prevent you from taking the proper action by answering the following questions:

What is your area of noncompliance?

Do you see this problem as serious?

What are the immediate consequences of your noncompliance?

What are the long-term consequences of your noncompliance?

How likely is it that these consequences will happen to you as opposed to other people who are similarly noncompliant?

What would you need to do to be compliant?

Is this regimen complex, or does it require you to make major changes in your daily routine?

In what ways will your adherence improve your health?

Do your family and friends think that it is important for you to comply with this regimen?

Does anyone remind you of your treatment and help you to adhere to it, or do those around you ignore or even discourage you?

How do you feel about the health care professional who recommended this treatment?

What role do these feelings play in your noncompliance?

How has this health care professional helped you to follow his or her recommendations? Has anything he or she has done discouraged you?

Do you feel that you are an active participant in your health care, or do you feel that you are following orders?

What could motivate you to be more compliant?

Answers

Fill in the Rest of the Story
I.   cognitive
I.A.   punishment; rewards (reinforcers)
I.B.   reciprocal; self-efficacy; cope
I.C.   intentions; attitudes; subjective; control
I.D.   precontemplation; maintenance, preparation; action; maintenance
II.   adhere
II.A.   cooperation
II.B.   person (patient); clinician (doctor);
II.C.   25; increases (improves); decreases (worsens)
III.A   severity; pain
III.B   increases; lower
III.C. barriers; women; single; stressful; lower; depression; more
III.D. income; social network (support network; supportive relationships; family)
III.E. physicians (Western health care providers); less
III.F. communication (relationship); decreases (falls); educational level; technical; female
III.G. small; interaction
IV.A.   understand; disappear (improve); optimistic; lifestyle (behavioral)
IV.B.   educational; more; Motivational; written; prompts (cues); contract

Multiple Choice

1. d	8. a	15. c	22. b
2. d	9. a	16. c	23. a
3. c	10. d	17. d	24. c
4. d	11. c	18. a	25. a
5. c	12. a	19. c	26. c
6. b	13. b	20. b	27. d
7. c	14. c	21. b	

Matching

1. i	2. d	3. g	4. h	5. a
6. f	7. b	8. c	9. e	

Good points to include in your essay answers:

1. A. Marissa has reached the maintenance stage, trying to maintain her changed behavior.
    B. To reach this last stage of the transtheoretical model, Marissa has passed through the other stages of this model.
        1. She first passed through the precontemplation stage in which she did not think about her sedentary lifestyle.

2. She then passed through the contemplation stage in which she considered adopting a more active lifestyle.
3. She has passed through the preparation stage in which she made preparations to exercise, such as deciding on what type of exercise to do and obtained the necessary equipment and clothing.
4. She has passed through the action stage because she began her program three weeks ago.

C. The transtheoretical model predicts that Marissa may cycle back into stages she has passed.
1. Marissa may relapse into a sedentary lifestyle.
2. If Marissa relapses, she may cycle back toward an active lifestyle.

2. A. Personality traits are not good predictors of compliance.
1. The noncompliant personality does not exist.
2. Situational factors are more important than personality.
B. Social circumstances are better predictors of compliance.
1. Economic factors show a relationship to compliance.
2. Social support for adherence increases compliance.
3. People whose cultural norms are consistent with the treatment tend to have higher compliance than those with different cultural values.

CHAPTER 5
Defining, Measuring, and Managing Stress

Learning Objectives

After studying Chapter 5, you should be able to

1. Explain how the nervous system and the endocrine system interact during the response to stress.
2. Compare Selye's theory of stress to Lazarus's theory of stress.
3. Compare the methods used to measure stress.
4. Describe the ways in which stress from cataclysmic events differs from life events.
5. Evaluate how daily hassles in the environment combine to produce stress.
6. Discuss the personal resources that affect coping.
7. Assess the effectiveness of personal coping strategies.
8. Evaluate relaxation training, cognitive behavioral therapy, and emotional disclosure for their effectiveness as stress management interventions.

Fill in the Rest of the Story

I.   The Nervous System and the Physiology of Stress

The nervous system is composed of nerve cells called _____ that provide internal communication by releasing chemical _____ that flow across the space between neurons called the _____ cleft. The nervous system is divided into two parts; the _____ _____ system consists of the brain and spinal cord, and all the other nerves in the body are in the _____ nervous system.

A. The Peripheral Nervous System

The peripheral nervous system is also divided into two divisions, the _____ nervous system, which activates voluntary muscles, and the _____ nervous system, which serves internal organs and glands. The autonomic nervous system (ANS) is divided into the _____ and

_____ divisions. The two main neurotransmitters of the ANS are

acetylcholine and _____.

B. The Neuroendocrine System

The endocrine system consists of ductless glands, and the _____

system consists of endocrine glands controlled by the nervous system. These glands release

_____ that travel through the blood and act on target organs. The

_____ gland is located in the brain and releases a number of hormones that

affect target organs in many parts of the body, including _____

hormone (ACTH), which acts on the adrenal glands. The _____ glands

are located on top of the kidneys and contain two structures that produce different

hormones, the _____ (outer covering) and the _____

(inner structure). The adrenal cortex secretes three types of hormones, including

glucocorticoids, the most important of which is _____. The adrenal

medulla is activated by the sympathetic nervous system and secretes catecholamines,

including _____ and _____.

C. The Physiology of the Stress Response

The stress reaction mobilizes body resources in emergency situations by activating the

_____ division of the _____ nervous system, which

is called the adrenomedullary response. The other route is through the hypothalamic-

pituitary-adrenal axis, resulting in the pituitary stimulating the adrenal cortex to produce

_____, including cortisol. Maintaining an appropriate level of activation

calls for varied levels of activation of the peripheral nervous system, which is a process

called _____. Prolonged activation of the sympathetic response produces

allostatic load, which may create problems.

II. Theories of Stress

Hans Selye and Richard Lazarus have proposed influential theories of stress.

A. Selye's View

Selye's theory defined stress as a generalized, or _____, response to a variety of environmental stressors. Selye hypothesized that the response to stress occurs in three stages, which taken together, are called the _____

_____ _____. These three stages are

_____, followed by resistance, and then _____. A criticism of Selye's theory is that it concentrates on the physiological and downplays the _____ aspects of stress.

B. Lazarus's View

Lazarus believed that people's perception of an event is more important than the event itself. His view is called _____ because it emphasizes the importance of the combination of psychological factors, such as cognitive mediation, appraisal, vulnerability, and coping. Lazarus recognized three kinds of appraisal—primary, secondary, and _____. A person's initial judgment of an event is _____ appraisal, whereas a person's perceived ability to cope with harm, threat, or challenge is _____ appraisal. Ongoing reevaluation of the situation is reappraisal. People who lack the resources to cope are _____. Their efforts to manage internal and external demands are called _____.

III. Measurement of Stress

The usefulness of stress measures rests on their ability to consistently predict some established criterion—for example, illness.

A. Methods of Measurement

Stress has been measured by several methods. Blood pressure, heart rate, galvanic skin response, respiration rate, and biochemical measures such as cortisol and catecholamine release are some of the _____ measures used to assess stress. A

73

disadvantage of these procedures is that the equipment and setting may themselves produce stress.

Most life events scales are patterned after the Holmes and Rahe _____

_____ _____ _____, which is based on the premise that any major change in life is stressful. Lazarus pioneered an alternative, a scale that measures _____ _____ rather than major life events. The Daily Hassles Scale assumes that only unpleasant events (hassles) can be stressful and emphasizes the perceived severity of the event. Lazarus and his colleagues also published the _____ Scale, which assumes that pleasant experiences will decrease stress. Another stress inventory is the Undergraduate Stress Questionnaire, a self-report scale that asks college students to check the items that have happened to them during the past two weeks. Most items are _____ rather than major life events.

B. Reliability and Validity of Stress Measures

The reliability of self-report stress inventories can be assessed by having a person fill out the inventory more than _____. The validity of stress inventories can be established by showing a relationship between scores on the inventory and

_____.

IV. Sources of Stress

Many sources of stress exist, and it is possible to organize them into cataclysmic events, life events, and daily hassles.

A. Cataclysmic Events

Cataclysmic events are unique and powerful, and these events affect large numbers of people. Cataclysmic events may be unintentional, such as natural disasters, or intentional acts, such as terrorist attacks or wars. Such events are more stressful when they are

_____. Some people who have experienced cataclysmic events develop

_____ _____ _____ (PTSD).

B. Life Events

Unlike _____ events, life events happen to everyone and require

people to adapt to the changes these events bring. These events affect _____

rather than groups and tend to take place across time rather than suddenly.

C. Daily Hassles

Daily hassles may arise from the physical or psychosocial environment. Physical

sources of stress include pollution, noise, crowding, and fear of crime, the combination of

which Eric Graig termed _____ _____. These hassles occur in

urban life but living in the "environment of _____" intensifies these

hassles. African Americans, other ethnic minorities, and women are the targets of

_____, which is one type of hassle that arises in the psychosocial

environment, both in the community and at work. Other stressors that affect people at work

include jobs that have high _____ and low _____. Work

may also produce stress when conflicts arise between work and _____

relationships.

Both women and men fulfill multiple roles as employee, spouse, and parent, but

_____ tend to perform more household work and child care chores, and

the demands may produce stress. Although relationships may be sources of conflict and

stress, they are also sources of support that help people _____ with stress.

V. Coping

_____ refers to strategies that people use to manage distress and

problems. Several resources influence coping.

A. Personal Resources That Influence Coping

The personal resource that includes the emotional quality of one's social contacts is

called _____ _____. Social support differs from

social contacts or _____ _____. The opposite of

social contacts is _____ _____. The Alameda

75

County Study indicated that as the number of social ties decreased, the death rate

_____. Social support may contribute to good health because (1)

people with good social support receive more encouragement and advice to seek

_____ care, (2) having a large social network may give people

confidence to cope with stressful situations, and (3) social support itself may provide a

_____ against disease.

A second personal resource is one's feelings of personal control. When people are

allowed to assume even small amounts of personal control and _____,

they seem to live longer and have healthier lives.

Kobasa's concept of the _____ personality hypothesizes some

highly stressed individuals remain healthy whereas others become

_____ because hardy individuals have a strong sense of

_____ to self, demonstrate an _____ locus of

control, and are likely to see necessary adjustments as a challenge.

B. Personal Coping Strategies

Productive coping aimed at changing the source of stress are called

_____-_____ coping, whereas emotion-focused coping, such

as drinking too much, may be oriented toward managing the emotions that accompany

stress. One coping strategy, _____ coping, allows people to take steps to

avoid an anticipated stressor. Problem-focused coping generally offers better outcomes, but

matching the coping strategy to the situation is the key to effective coping.

VI. Behavioral Interventions for Managing Stress

Behavioral techniques may be seen as alternative or mind-body medicine, but

psychologists concentrate on the behavioral aspects and consider them part of psychology.

A. Relaxation Training

Relaxation techniques are important interventions to manage stress. These techniques

include progressive _____ relaxation and autogenics training. With

_____ muscle relaxation, clients learn to relax the entire body, one

muscle group at a time, and to breathe deeply and exhale slowly. _____ training

consists of exercises to achieve _____ and instructions to change thought processes.

Relaxation is an effective method of coping with stress.

B. Cognitive Behavioral Therapy

Cognitive behavioral therapy (_____) draws from _____

_____ in accepting that cognitions are an important basis for behavior and

from _____ _____ in applying principles of reinforcement to

change behavior.

Donald Meichenbaum and Roy Cameron developed a cognitive behavioral strategy for

managing stress called stress _____ training, which includes three

stages: (1) a reconceptualization stage where patients are encouraged to

_____ differently about their stress or pain experiences, (2) an

acquisition and _____ of skills stage where patients are taught relaxation

and controlled breathing skills, and a (3) _____-

_____ stage where patients apply their coping skills to their daily

environment. Research has supported the effectiveness of stress inoculation and other

cognitive behavioral therapies for managing stress.

C. Emotional Disclosure

James Pennebaker and his associates have demonstrated the therapeutic value of

expression their strong _____ by talking or _____

about the traumatic events. Emotional disclosure is different from emotional

_____, which involves emotional outbursts or emotional venting,

such as crying, laughing, yelling, or throwing objects. Emotional disclosure, in contrast,

involves the transfer of emotions into _____ and thus requires a

measure of self-reflection. Emotional disclosure has brought about a number of positive

physiological changes, as well as psychological and behavioral changes.

Multiple Choice Questions

_____ 1. A neuron is a(n)
   a. neurotransmitter.
   b. individual nerve cell.
   c. synapse.
   d. none of the above.

_____ 2. The synaptic cleft is
   a. a neuron.
   b. an individual nerve cell.
   c. the space between neurons.
   d. a group of ganglions.
   e. none of the above.

_____ 3. The brain and the spinal cord are considered to be
   a. the peripheral nervous system.
   b. the central nervous system.
   c. the cardiovascular system.
   d. the somatic nervous system.

_____ 4. The two sub-divisions of the autonomic nervous system are
   a. sympathetic and parasympathetic nervous systems.
   b. the brain and the spinal cord.
   c. central and peripheral.
   d. afferents and efferents.

_____ 5. The adrenal glands are part of the _____ system.
   a. nervous
   b. cardiovascular
   c. digestive
   d. endocrine

_____ 6. The "fight or flight" response is mediated through the
   a. central nervous system.
   b. sympathetic nervous system.
   c. parasympathetic nervous system.
   d. somatic nervous system.

_____ 7. Selye viewed stress as
   a. a cognitive function.
   b. a nonspecific response.
   c. a specific response.
   d. none of the above.

_____ 8. Which of these is a stage of the General Adaptation Syndrome?
a. the alarm stage
b. the illness stage
c. death
d. self-efficacy

_____ 9. Which of the following has been a criticism of Selye's theory of stress?
a. The theory places too much emphasis on emotional and psychological factors.
b. The theory ignores physiological factors that underlie the stress response.
c. The theory places too much emphasis on appraisal and too little on coping.
d. The theory places too much emphasis on physiological factors and too little on psychological factors.

_____ 10. The theorist who emphasized psychological and cognitive factors in stress was
a. Hans Selye.
b. Walter Cannon.
c. Richard Lazarus.
d. none of the above.

_____ 11. Which of these was NOT listed by Lazarus and Folkman as being part of a person's ability to cope with an event?
a. problem-solving ability
b. the magnitude of the event itself
c. material resources, such as money
d. belief that one can cope with the event

_____ 12. A vulnerable person, according to Lazarus,
a. lacks the ability to rationalize stressful situations.
b. lacks the resources to cope with an important event.
c. is already ill but has not yet been diagnosed.
d. has too much ability to cope with stressful events.

_____ 13. Health psychologists are most likely to use which type of instrument to measure stress?
a. performance tests
b. physiological measures
c. self-report scales
d. reports of significant others

_____ 14. What scale assumes that changes in life adjustment are the key factor in measuring stress?
a. the Social Readjustment Rating Scale
b. the Daily Hassles Scale
c. the Uplift Scale
d. the Perceived Stress Scale

_____ 15. When Kyle filled out the Holmes and Rahe Social Readjustment Rating Scale, his score was 500. Such a score indicates that Kyle
    a. has a decreased risk for a stress-related disorder.
    b. will develop a disease during the next year.
    c. will develop a psychological disorder during the next year.
    d. has more stress than most people.

_____ 16. Which scale emphasizes the importance of everyday events?
    a. the Social Readjustment Rating Scale
    b. the revised Daily Hassles and Uplifts Scale
    c. the Perceived Stress Scale
    d. all of the above

_____ 17. One way of determining the reliability of a stress inventory is to have people fill out the inventory twice. Another method is to compare participants' scores with
    a. scores of spouses who filled out the inventory from the participant's point of view.
    b. the number of illnesses per person per year.
    c. scores on the Social Readjustment Rating Scale.
    d. the number of people who take the stress inventory.

_____ 18. The validity of self-report inventories is complicated by what question?
    a. What should the scale measure?
    b. How high should the reliability be?
    c. What psychological factors underlie the stress response?
    d. What physiological factors underlie stress?

_____ 19. The MOST important attribute of a stress inventory is its
    a. reliability.
    b. ability to test hypothetical assumptions underlying a given theory of stress.
    c. standardization.
    d. ability to predict illness.

_____ 20. Cataclysmic events such as earthquakes and hurricanes may not be as traumatic as cataclysmic events such as terrorist attacks because
    a. more people are affected by terrorist attacks.
    b. news coverage is higher for terrorist attacks than for natural disasters.
    c. terrorist attacks affect individuals and not entire families.
    d. the intention to cause harm makes events more stressful.

_____ 21. Life events are stressful because
    a. they produce change and require adaptation.
    b. they introduce negative events into people's lives.
    c. they endanger people's lives.
    d. they produce higher levels of vulnerability than hassles do.

_____ 22. Urban press refers to
   a. city dwellers' flight to the suburbs.
   b. the many sources of environmental stressors that affect city living.
   c. campaigns by city newspapers that emphasize the healthy environment of the city.
   d. health-related news reports carried by the mass media.

_____ 23. In comparing crowding and density, Stokols proposed that
   a. crowding is physical and density is psychological.
   b. crowding is psychological and density is physical.
   c. both crowding and density are psychological.
   d. both crowding and density are physical.

_____ 24. During a recent basketball game, 27,000 people were in attendance. That many people in a relatively small environment would constitute
   a. overcrowding.
   b. crowding.
   c. a riot.
   d. density.

_____ 25. Discrimination is often a source of stress for
   a. African Americans.
   b. Hispanic Americans.
   c. women
   d. all of these people.

_____ 26. With regard to crime, which of these statements is most accurate?
   a. All categories of crime are on the increase in the United States.
   b. Fear of crime is related more to media attention than to crime incidence.
   c. Firearm homicide rates are decreasing.
   d. Homicide and robbery rates are sharply increasing.

_____ 27. Which of these factors could be a source of stress?
   a. family relations
   b. crowding
   c. multiple roles
   d. neighborhood crime
   e. all of the above

_____ 28. Stress-related illnesses are LEAST common among
   a. people who have jobs with high demands and low levels of control.
   b. people who have jobs with high demands and high levels of control.
   c. waiters and waitresses.
   d. construction workers.

_____ 29. Which of these jobs is probably MOST stressful?
   a. college professor
   b. restaurant owner
   c. farmer
   d. food service work

_____ 30. Florence feels emotional concern from her husband, who also provides instrumental aid and communicates love and affection to Florence. Thus, Florence receives _____ from her husband.
   a. a social network
   b. social support
   c. unconditional positive regard
   d. agape

_____ 31. An absence of social relationships best describes
   a. social network.
   b. social isolation.
   c. sociopathy.
   d. socioeconomic deficiency.

_____ 32. A study by Ellen Langer and Judith Rodin of nursing home residents showed that elderly people were more likely to remain healthy if
   a. they had plants in their rooms.
   b. they exercised even small amounts of personal control.
   c. their caregivers rearranged their room furniture on a regular basis.
   d. they received daily letters from their friends and family.

_____ 33. Which of these factors is NOT an element of the hardy personality?
   a. compromise
   b. commitment
   c. control
   d. challenge

_____ 34. What do psychologists call those strategies that people use to manage the distressing problems in their lives?
   a. defense mechanisms
   b. external controls
   c. protective devices
   d. coping techniques

_____ 35. Strategies aimed at changing a person's source of stress are called
   a. fear control techniques.
   b. problem-focused coping.
   c. emotion-focused coping.
   d. emotional venting.

_____ 36. When Damon was fired from his job, he escalated his drinking from two drinks a day to 10 or 12. His reaction to losing his job would be called
   a. sublimation.
   b. problem-focused coping.
   c. a reaction formation.
   d. emotion-focused coping.

_____ 37. What relaxation technique involves patients reclining in a comfortable chair with no distracting lights or sounds, breathing slowly, and learning to relax different muscle groups?
   a. progressive muscle relaxation
   b. rational emotive therapy
   c. hypnosuggestive therapy
   d. guided imagery

_____ 38. Health psychologists are most likely to use relaxation training to help people
   a. cope with stress-related problems.
   b. determine their level of pain.
   c. solve marital and other interpersonal problems.
   d. change unhealthy eating habits.

_____ 39. An approach to behavior management that includes both a method for changing thoughts or attitudes and behavior meets the definition of
   a. reinforcement therapy.
   b. biofeedback
   c. cognitive behavioral therapy.
   d. motivational interviewing.

_____ 40. How effective is stress inoculation training? Stress inoculation training
   a. is no more effective than a placebo.
   b. is effective in altering anxiety but not in increasing performance under stress.
   c. is effective in increasing performance under stress but not in decreasing anxiety.
   d. is effective both in decreasing anxiety and in increasing performance under stress.

_____ 41. When psychologists say that emotional expression improves psychological and physical health, they are referring to
   a. writing or talking about traumatic events.
   b. crying or yelling.
   c. the confession of wrongs that one has done.
   d. any of the above, all of which would be emotional expression and produce health benefits.

_____ 42. James Pennebaker and his associates found that people who survived traumatic experiences achieved better physical health if they
a. blocked those experiences from conscious thought.
b. wrote or talked about those experiences.
c. were children when they experienced trauma.
d. were at least 50 years old when they experienced the trauma.

Key Terms

Define each of the following:

adrenocortical response —

adrenomedullary response —

autonomic nervous system —

cognitive behavioral therapy —

crowding —

daily hassles —

emotion-focused coping —

general adaptation syndrome —

hormones —

life events —

neurotransmitters —

parasympathetic nervous system —

posttraumatic stress disorder (PTSD) —

proactive coping —

problem-focused coping —

progressive muscle relaxation —

social support —

stress inoculation —

sympathetic nervous system —

urban press —

vulnerability —

Matching

Match the following:

1. synaptic cleft   a. transactional view

2. proactive coping   b. epinephrine

3. social support   c. buffer against stress

4. glucocorticoid   d. therapeutic benefit of writing about traumatic
                                         experiences

5. catecholamine   e. space between neurons

6. Selye   f. can prevent stress

7. Lazarus   g. general adaptation syndrome

8. sympathetic nervous system   h. cortisol

9. James Pennebaker   i. factors that make city living stressful

10. urban press   j. autonomic division

1. _____ 2. _____ 3. _____ 4. _____ 5. _____

6. _____ 7. _____ 8. _____ 9. _____ 10. _____

Physiology of the Stress Response

Fill in the blanks to complete the correct responses for the neuroendocrine and autonomic nervous system activation during stress.

In the brain

_____ gland

neuroendocrine

autonomic
nervous system

ACTH

stimulates

_____

division

Adrenal _____

secretes _____

and

Adrenal _____

secretes _____

and

_____

_____ pupils in eye

_____ heartbeat

_____ stomach activity

_____ blood pressure

_____ respiration

_____ muscle strength

Essay Questions

1. Franklin is a college sophomore majoring in premed. He has made 67% on his first exam in anatomy. Analyze Franklin's response to this event in terms of Lazarus's theory of stress, including appraisal and vulnerability.

2. Discuss personal resources and how they affect a person's ability to cope with stress.

3. Outline some coping strategies for Franklin, the college premed major who received a bad grade on his first anatomy exam, and discuss how useful behavioral interventions would be for him.

Let's Get Personal— Assess Your Stress

You can assess your stress by taking the Undergraduate Stress Questionnaire, which appears as the Check Your Health Risks box at the beginning of this chapter. Fill it out and add your stress points to determine your score.

Do you think that the USQ captured the stresses of your life?

What questions were inappropriate for you?

What areas of stress did the USQ miss?

Do you think that a stress inventory such as the Social Readjustment Rating Scale would be more or less appropriate?

Answers

Fill in the Rest of the Story

I.   neurons; neurotransmitters; synaptic; central nervous; peripheral

I.A.   somatic; autonomic; sympathetic; parasympathetic; norepinephrine

I.B.   neuroendocrine; hormones; pituitary; adrenocorticotropic; adrenal; cortex; medulla; cortisol; epinephrine; norepinephrine

I.C.   sympathetic; autonomic; glucocorticoids; allostasis

II.A.   nonspecific; General Adaptation Syndrome; alarm; exhaustion; psychological

II.B.   transactional; reappraisal; primary; secondary; vulnerable; coping

III.A. physiological; Social Readjustment Rating Scale; daily (everyday) hassles; Uplifts; hassles

III.B. once; illness (health)

IV.A.   intentional; posttraumatic stress disorder

IV.B.   cataclysmic; individuals

IV.C.   urban press; poverty; discrimination; demands; control; personal (family); women; cope

V.   Coping

V.A.   social support; social networks; social isolation; increased; medical; buffer; responsibility; hardiness; ill; commitment; internal

V.B.   problem-focused; proactive

VI.A.   muscle; progressive; Autogenics; relaxation

VI.B.   CBT; cognitive therapy; behavior therapy (behavior modification); inoculation; think; rehearsal; follow-through

VI.C.   emotions; writing; expression (catharsis); language (words)

Multiple Choice

1.	b	10.	c	18.	a	26.	b	34.	d
2.	c	11.	b	19.	d	27.	e	35.	b
3.	b	12.	b	20.	d	28.	b	36.	d
4.	a	13.	c	21.	a	29.	d	37.	a
5.	d	14.	a	22.	b	30.	b	38.	a
6.	b	15.	d	23.	b	31.	b	39.	c
7.	b	16.	b	24.	d	32.	b	40.	d
8.	a	17.	a	25.	d	33.	a	41.	a
9.	d							42.	b

Matching

1.	e	2.	f	3.	c	4.	h	5.	b
6.	g	7.	a	8.	j	9.	d	10.	i

Good points to include in your essay answers:

1. A. Franklin would go through the process of appraisal, including primary and secondary appraisal, and reappraisal.
    1. His primary appraisal would be his initial perception of the low grade in terms of stressful, irrelevant, or benign-positive. A primary appraisal of *stressful* is likely because Franklin would probably perceive a low grade as harmful, threatening, or challenging to his current grade point average and thus to his future career.
    2. Franklin's secondary appraisal would include his evaluation of his ability to cope with the low grade. He might consider how many other tests and how well he thinks he can do on other work for the course.
    3. Reappraisal includes reevaluations of the situation, which may decrease or increase stress. Franklin may experience reduced stress if he finds that others in the class also did poorly, leading the instructor to "curve" the grades. His stress might be increased by good performance by his classmates or by the importance of this exam for his final grade.
    B. Franklin's vulnerability will be determined by his perception of his ability to cope with the grade.
    1. He may feel vulnerable and stressed because he studied and believes that he did as well as he can.
    2. He may feel less vulnerable because he believes that he can improve his grade.

2. A. Social support is important for health and longevity.
    1. The Alameda County Study showed that social support is positively related to low mortality rate.
    2. Social support may affect health by
       a. Providing encouragement for adopting healthy behaviors or seeking medical care.
       b. Helping people cope with stress.
       c. Altering the physiological response to stress.
       d. Buffering against stress.
    B. Personal control is also important for health.
    1. People who have control over the important aspects of their lives have an internal locus of control, which is generally healthier than an external locus of control.
    2. Studies on nursing home residents by Langer and Rodin demonstrated that even a small degree of personal control can be beneficial to health and lower mortality.
    C. According to the concept of the hardy personality, some people are more able to cope than others.
    1. Such individuals have a strong sense of commitment, have an internal locus of control, and see adaptation and adjustments as challenges rather than as stressors.
    2. People with the characteristics of the hardy personality are less likely than others to develop stress-related illnesses.

3. A. Franklin may seek social support in order to feel better, but this coping strategy is not his best choice.
    B. Franklin needs to choose some problem-focused strategies to improve his grades.
    1. Franklin should analyze his situation to determine the reason for his bad grade and then take action to change the situation.

2. If he did not study enough, one strategy would be to make a schedule to allow more time for studying.

3. If he did not understand the material, he might seek the help of his instructor, find a tutor, or form a study group to give him social support and the knowledge and resources of other students to help with studying.

C. Franklin may choose to consider proactive coping to prevent this problem from occurring in future semesters.

D. Franklin might profit from any of the behavioral management approaches, but Franklin's situation does not seem appropriate to emotional disclosure.

1. Relaxation could help him to cope with the many demands of student life and concentrate on studying.

2. Cognitive behavioral therapy could help Franklin re-evaluate his situation and learn new skills to deal with his situation.

CHAPTER 6
Understanding Stress and Disease

Learning Objectives

After studying Chapter 6, you should be able to

1. Describe the organs and function of the immune system.
2. Explain how the field of psychoneuroimmunology has established a link between stress and disease.
3. Evaluate the diathesis-stress model and its explanation of the relationship between stress and disease.
4. Evaluate the role that stress plays in headaches, infectious disease, cardiovascular disease, diabetes, and depression.

Fill in the Rest of the Story

I. Physiology of the Immune System

The immune system consists of tissues, organs, and processes that protect the body from invasion by foreign material such as bacteria, _____, and fungi. It also removes worn-out or damaged cells from the body.

A. Organs of the Immune System

The immune system includes lymph, a circulating fluid that contains a type of white blood cell called _____. Various types of lymphocytes include T-cells, B-cells, and _____ _____ (NK) cells.

B. Function of the Immune System

The immune system defends the body against foreign invaders through both specific and nonspecific responses. Specific immunity is called _____-_____ immunity, and those substances manufactured in response to a specific invader are called _____. After the invaders have been destroyed, the immune system keeps the critical information that allows future manufacture of antibodies, creating _____ to the invader, which can persist for years.

C. Immune System Disorders

Examples of the immune system's failure to protect a person include acquired immune deficiency syndrome (AIDS), allergies, and _____ disorders that originate from the immune system's failure to distinguish body cells from invaders and results in an attack on one's own body cells.

II. Psychoneuroimmunology

The interdisciplinary field that focuses on the interactions among behavior, the nervous system, the endocrine system, and the immune system is called _____. Research in psychoneuroimmunology has attempted to reveal the interactions among behavior, the _____ system, the _____ system, and the immune system by demonstrating that behavior can affect the immune system and that illness can result from these effects.

A. History of Psychoneuroimmunology

In 1975, Robert Ader and Nicholas Cohen demonstrated that the immune system could be _____ and thus began the field of psychoneuroimmunology.

B. Research in Psychoneuroimmunology

Research has demonstrated that behavior can _____ immune system function, and depressed immune system function relates to subsequent _____. Research in the field of psychoneuroimmunology has demonstrated the sequence of _____, immune system depression, and disease.

C. Physical Mechanisms of Influence

The link between behavior and depressed immune function must occur through some physical mechanism. Researchers have looked at both the action of the peripheral nervous system during stress and neuroendocrine responses in the _____. The immune system also produces _____, chemical messengers that signal the nervous system. Therefore, many possibilities exist for mechanisms of influence.

III. Does Stress Cause Disease?

Stress is one of many factors that may cause illness, but in general, most people who experience stress will _____ develop a disease.

A. The Diathesis-Stress Model

The diathesis-stress model offers a possible answer to the question of why some stressed people get _____ whereas others are unaffected by _____. This model suggests that some individuals are _____ to stress-related diseases because either genetic weakness or biochemical imbalance inherently predisposes them to those diseases. Whether inherited or _____, the vulnerability to stress-related disease is relatively permanent. For people with a strong predisposition to a disease, even a mild environmental stressor may be sufficient to produce _____.

B. Stress and Disease

Because stress responses can act in many ways throughout the body, these responses have the potential to cause _____ damage and contribute to such disorders as headaches, infectious diseases, cardiovascular disease, and other physiological illnesses. Stress may contribute to both tension and _____ headaches, the two most common types of headache.

Research that involved exposing people to _____ viruses has shown that stress is an important factor in vulnerability to infectious illness.

The relationship between stress and cardiovascular disease is complex and not well-established. Stress has a stronger influence on temporary increases in blood pressure than on chronic hypertension. The tendency for some people to react more strongly than other people to stress is called _____, and the tendency to react more strongly to stressors is higher for African Americans than for European Americans. This

97

ethnic difference may relate to a higher rate of _____

_____ for African Americans. Stress is not the primary underlying cause

for most _____; rather, the bacterium *H. pylori* is responsible. Stress may also be

implicated in physiological disorders such as Type 1 and Type 2

_____, asthma, rheumatoid, and arthritis.

C. Stress and Psychological Disorders

Stress may also relate to a number of psychological disorders, including depression and

anxiety, although the evidence for such a causal link is not strong. Although depressed

people may report more negative _____ _____ than do

nondepressed people, little or no evidence supports a causal relationship. However, the

tendency to _____ over problems increases the risk for depression, and

several type of chronic stress also relate to the development of _____.

Anxiety disorders include panic attacks, agoraphobia, generalized anxiety, obsessive-

compulsive disorders, and _____ _____ disorder

(PTSD). PTSD is, by definition, related to stress, but stress is less clearly related to the

other anxiety disorders.

Multiple Choice Questions

_____ 1. The main function of the _____ system is to defend the body against foreign
invaders.
   a. endocrine
   b. autonomic nervous
   c. somatic nervous
   d. immune

_____ 2. Which of these is an organ of the immune system?
   a. liver
   b. heart
   c. tonsils
   d. bronchi

_____ 3. If the body were a kingdom, the immune system would be the
    a. king.
    b. court jester.
    c. army.
    d. heir to the throne.

_____ 4. The function of antibodies is to
    a. create leukocytes.
    b. produce immunity.
    c. promote memory T-cells.
    d. divide T-cells from B-cells.

_____ 5. HIV is caused by
    a. homosexuality.
    b. injection drug use.
    c. a virus.
    d. a bacterium.
    e. all of the above.

_____ 6. Psychoneuroimmunology is a relatively new discipline dealing primarily with
    a. the causes of HIV.
    b. the cure for AIDS.
    c. the interactions among behavior, the endocrine system, the immune system, and the nervous system.
    d. the interactions among behavior, the cardiovascular system, the immune system, the nervous system, and stress.

_____ 7. Immune system function can be decreased by
    a. people writing about their traumatic experiences.
    b. arguments with spouses.
    c. final exams.
    d. both b and c
    e. all of the above.

_____ 8. The notion that some people are more inherently vulnerable to the effects of stress than are other people is called
    a. the hardiness hypothesis.
    b. the identity disruption model.
    c. psychoneuroimmunology.
    d. the diathesis-stress model.

_____ 9. If stress causes illness, then what system most likely plays a central role in that process?
    a. nervous system
    b. digestive system
    c. cardiovascular system
    d. immune system

_____10. Evidence is most clear for a relationship between stress and
    a. ulcers.
    b. Alzheimer's disease.
    c. decreased immune function.
    d. cancer.
    e. asthma.

_____11. The types of stress related to tension and migraine headache are those that are best measured by _____ scales.
    a. daily hassles
    b. daily uplifts
    c. life events
    d. diathesis

_____12. When Sheldon Cohen intentionally exposed people to respiratory viruses, he found that people
    a. with an inherent vulnerability to stress were the ones most likely to develop an infectious disease.
    b. most stressed prior to the exposure were the ones most likely to develop an infectious disease.
    c. least stressed prior to the exposure were the ones most likely to develop an infectious disease.
    d. with a hardy personality developed fewer infectious diseases than other people.

_____13. The term *reactivity* means that some people
    a. respond more strongly to stress than do other people.
    b. respond with more intense anger than do other people.
    c. respond more quickly to fearful stimuli than do other people.
    d. all of the above.

_____14. A large international study on risk factors for heart attack showed that
    a. a variety of stressors are related to increased risk for heart attack.
    b. stressors increased the risk for heart attack for men but not for women.
    c. financial stress but not workplace stress increase the risk.
    d. no relationship appeared for stress, but income level was an important predictor.

_____15. What relationship does stress have with diabetes?
    a. Stress is related to the development of Type 1 diabetes but not to Type 2 diabetes.
    b. Stress is related to the management of Type 1 diabetes but not to its development.
    c. Stress is related to the development and management of both Type 1 and Type 2 diabetes.
    d. Stress shows little relationship to either type of diabetes.

_____16. Which of the following increases the risk for depression?
   a. genetic vulnerability
   b. a negative outlook and the tendency to dwell on problems
   c. a large family
   d. both a and b
   e. all of the above

_____17. The immune system produces _____ that seem to be related to the development of depression.
   a. neurotransmitters
   b. neurohormones
   c. proinflammatory cytokines
   d. leucocytes

_____18. Research suggests that the strongest association is between stress and
   a. depression.
   b. anxiety.
   c. infectious illnesses.
   d. mood.

_____19. Research on the effect of stress on depression suggests that
   a. people with the ability to cope with stress suffer very few depressive symptoms.
   b. stress by itself typically results in severe depression.
   c. stress is a necessary condition for depression.
   d. stress is the trigger for more than half of all depressive episodes.

_____20 Health psychologists are most confident that
   a. stress is the primary risk factor for cardiovascular disease.
   b. stress can trigger an asthma attack.
   c. stress is the primary cause of trait anxiety.
   d. no relationship exists between stress and depression.

_____21. Stress, by definition, is associated with
   a. asthma.
   b. agoraphobia.
   c. posttraumatic stress disorder.
   d. state anxiety.

_____22. Charlotte suffers from recurrent memories that intrude into her thoughts. She also has unpleasant dreams that replay a distressing experienced of being mugged and robbed three years ago. The extreme psychological and physiological distress she experiences best fits the definition of
   a. posttraumatic stress disorder.
   b. clinical depression.
   c. schizophrenia.
   d. trait anxiety.

_____23. Contrary to popular belief, stress is a minor factor in the development of
   a. rheumatoid arthritis.
   b. headache.
   c. asthma.
   d. ulcers.

_____24. Stress during pregnancy is most likely to result in
   a. spontaneous abortions.
   b. underweight babies.
   c. multiple births.
   d. all of the above.

_____25. The person who is most likely to experience a stress-related disorder is one who
   a. has a diathesis that protects against stress.
   b. experiences lowered levels of immune system function.
   c. has an executive position that requires many decisions.
   d. has relatives who have experienced stress-related disorders during adolescence.

_____26. Garland has been healthy for the past year. What does his good health reveal about his level of stress?
   a. He has a low level of stress.
   b. He has a high level of stress but good coping abilities.
   c. He has a supportive wife who provides a relationship in which he can be emotionally expressive.
   d. Nothing definite—the relationship between stress and illness is far from perfect.

Key Terms

Define each of the following:

AIDS —

antigens —

cytokines —

immunity —

lymphatic system —

lymphocytes —

psychoneuroimmunology —

PTSD —

rheumatoid arthritis —

T-cells —

Matching

Match the following:

1. Robert Ader and Nicholas Cohen
   a. nonspecific immune response

2. T-cells and B-cells
   b. demonstrated that stress plays a role in vulnerability to infectious illness

3. antibodies
   c. demonstrated that immune response is lowered by psychological stress

4. Janice Kiecolt-Glaser and Ronald Glaser
   d. holds that some people are more vulnerable to stress than others

5. Sheldon Cohen
   e. demonstrated that the immune system can be classically conditioned

6. phagocytosis
   f. lymphocytes

7. autoimmune disorders
   g. specific immune response

8. thymus and tonsils
   h. organs of the immune system

9. diathesis-stress model
   i. psychological disorder caused by stress

10. posttraumatic stress disorder
    j. failure to distinguish body cells from invaders

1. _____ 2. _____ 3. _____ 4. _____ 5. _____

6. _____ 7. _____ 8. _____ 9. _____ 10. _____

Understanding the Immune Response

Fill in the missing information to complete the sequence of events for the primary immune response. How does the time frame compare to that of the secondary immune response?

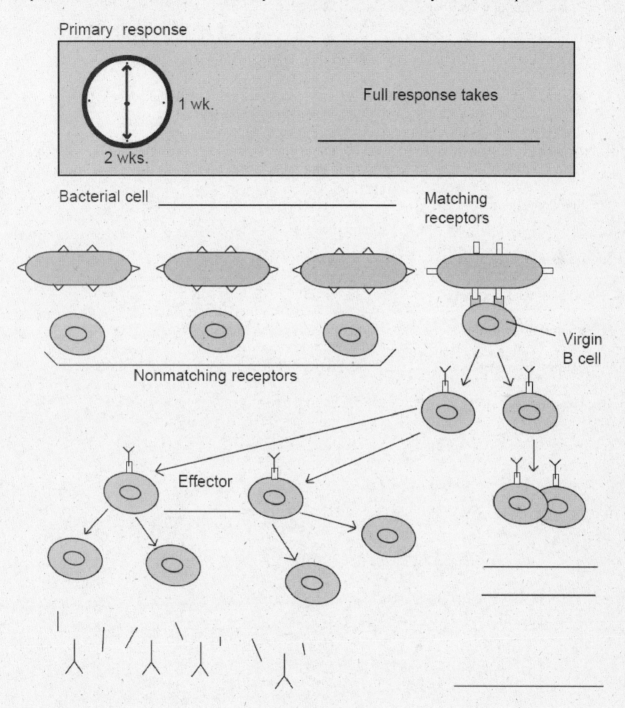

Primary response

1 wk.

2 wks.

Full response takes

_____

Bacterial cell _____ Matching receptors

Nonmatching receptors

Virgin B cell

Effector

_____

105

Essay Questions

1. What happens when the immune system begins to lose its effectiveness? How can this loss occur?

2. Which physical illnesses have a strong stress component? For which is the evidence less clear?

Let's Get Personal — Headache Analysis

Do you have headaches that relate to the stress in your life? Headaches are the disorder with the strongest relationship to stress, and most people experience headaches at some times Tension, migraine, and cluster headaches all have some stress component.

To analyze the relationship between your stress and headaches, keep a headache diary for at least a week. Note your headaches, time of day, and activities that preceded each one. To what extent did some stressful event or combination of events trigger the headaches? How did you cope with your headaches, and did these coping techniques address the stress component?

For each day and for each headache, furnish the following information:

Time of headache—

What I was doing when I noticed I had a headache—

Was stress a factor in this triggering this headache?

If so, what was the stressful event?

What I did when I noticed I had a headache—

This action worked to alleviate my headache by—

Answers

Fill in the Rest of the Story

I.   viruses
I.A.   lymphocytes; natural killer
I.B.   cell-mediated; antibodies; immunity
I.C.   autoimmune
II.   psychoneuroimmunology; endocrine; nervous
II.A.   conditioned
II.B.   depress; disease (illness); behavior
II.C.   brain; cytokines
III.   not
III.A. sick; stress; vulnerable, acquired; illness (disease)
III.B. physiological (organic); migraine; respiratory (cold or rhino); reactivity; cardiovascular disease; ulcers; diabetes
III.C. life events; ruminate; depression; posttraumatic stress

Multiple Choice

1. d	8. d	14. a	21. c
2. c	9. d	15. c	22. a
3. c	10. c	16. d	23. d
4. b	11. a	17. c	24. b
5. c	12 b	18. c	25. b
6. c	13. a	19. a	26. d
7. d		20. b	

Matching

1. e	2. f	3. g	4. c	5. b
6. a	7. j	8. h	9. d	10. i

Good points to include in your essay answers:

1. A. When the immune system loses its effectiveness, the body becomes vulnerable to a wide variety of viral, bacterial, fungal, and parasitic invaders.
    1. Impairment of nonspecific immune function blocks tissue repair, because inflammation and phagocytosis will not occur, leaving the body vulnerable to infection by these invaders.
    2. Impairment of specific immune functions decreases the formation of antibodies, which attack specific invaders; this deficit prevents the formation of immunity.

3. With impaired immune system function, attempts at immunization could be dangerous, because immunization typically occurs through the introduction of weakened forms of the disease; without the ability to form antibodies, these weakened pathogens could cause disease.

B. Immune deficiency occurs both as an inherent condition and as the result of infection with the human immunodeficiency virus.

1. Children who fail to develop functional immune systems must remain isolated from pathogens, or they will die from exposure to the many diseases that most people can withstand.
2. People infected with HIV lose their immune function and die from one of the many nfections that their bodies can no longer fight.

2. A. Stress is a factor in both vascular and tension headaches.
   B. Stress is related to vulnerability to infectious illness.
   C. The relationship between stress and cardiovascular disease is not straightforward, but ome people show high levels of reactivity or sodium retention when under stress, which ay be a factor in the development of cardiovascular disease.
   D. Stress is not the underlying cause of ulcers; *H. pylori* infection is present in over 90% of lcer cases.
   E. Other disorders such as diabetes, premature delivery in pregnancy, asthma, and heumatoid arthritis are related to stress, but the exact role of stress in the development of hese diseases is not clear.
   F. Evidence exists that stress is related to physical disorders, but the evidence is less clear han most people assume.

CHAPTER 7
Understanding and Managing Pain

Learning Objectives

After studying Chapter 7, you should be able to

1. Explain how the nervous system registers pain.
2. Discuss the role of neurotransmitters and proinflammatory cytokines in the experience of pain.
3. Identify and discuss the three stages of pain.
4. Describe what factors influence the variability in the experience of pain.
5. Evaluate the theories that explain pain.
6. Identify and evaluate the methods for assessing pain.
7. Describe pain syndromes such as headache, low back pain, arthritis pain, cancer pain, and phantom limb pain.
8. Discuss the effectiveness and limitations of medical treatments for pain.
9. Evaluate the effectiveness of pain management using relaxation training, behavior modification, cognitive therapy, and cognitive behavioral therapy.

Fill in the Rest of the Story

I. Pain and the Nervous System

All sensory stimulation, including pain, starts with activation of sensory neurons and proceeds with the relay of neural impulses toward the _____.

A. Somatosensory System

The _____ system conveys sensory information from the body through the spinal cord to the brain. Sensory, or _____, neurons convey information from sense organs toward the brain. Primary afferents are those neurons that have receptors in the sense organs. The vast number of neurons and their interconnections makes neural transmission complex.

Neurons that transmit pain messages are called _____. Three different types

of neurons are involved with transmitting pain impulses. The large _____-

_____ fibers and smaller A-delta fibers are covered with a protective covering

called _____, which speeds neural transmission. The smaller and more

common _____ fibers require high levels of stimulation to fire.

B. The Spinal Cord

Primary afferents from the skin enter the _____ _____

where they synapse with secondary afferents called _____ cells in the

dorsal horns of the spinal cord. The dorsal horns contain several layers called

_____, and laminae 1 and 2 form a structure called the

_____ _____ that receives sensory input from the A

and C fibers. Complex interactions of sensory input occur in the laminae of the dorsal horns,

and these interactions may affect the perception of sensory input before it gets to the brain.

C. The Brain

The brain structure that receives sensory input from the different neural tracts in the

spinal cord is the _____. The skin is mapped in the somatosensory cortex

in the _____ lobe of the cerebral cortex, and the proportion of cortex

devoted to an area of skin is proportional to that skin's sensitivity to stimulation. Sensory

information from internal organs are not mapped as precisely as the skin.

D. Neurotransmitters and Pain

The neurotransmitters that form the basis for neural transmission also play a role in pain

perception. The discovery of the endogenous opiates—enkephalin, _____,

and dynorphin—led to the discovery of neural receptors specialized for these

neurotransmitters and the conclusion that opiate drugs produce analgesia because of the brain's own chemistry. The neurotransmitters glutamate and substance P and the chemicals bradykinin and prostaglandins may increase pain perception. _____

_____ produced by the immune system are also involved in pain.

E. The Modulation of Pain

When a structure in the midbrain is stimulated, pain relief occurs. This structure is called the _____ _____. The neurons in the periaqueductal gray synapse with neurons in a structure in the medulla called the _____

_____ _____. These neurons descend to the spinal cord and may constitute a descending control system for pain perception.

II. The Meaning of Pain

Pain consists of sensations and reactions to those sensations, producing a physical and an emotional component.

A. Definition of Pain

The International Association for the Study of Pain defined pain as "an unpleasant sensory and _____ experience associated with actual or potential tissue damage, or described in terms of such damage." At least three stages of pain have been identified. The type of pain that is ordinarily adaptive and lasts a relatively short period of time is _____ pain. It includes pain from cuts, burns, and other physical trauma. _____ pain endures beyond the time of normal healing, is relatively constant, is often reinforced by other people, and becomes self-perpetuating. Pain experienced between acute and chronic pain is called _____. This intermediate time is critical because during this time the pain may either terminate or evolve into chronic pain.

B. The Experience of Pain

The experience of wounded soldiers during World War II showed that injury could occur without pain, which demonstrates that situational factors influence the experience of pain. In addition, _____ factors are an influence; people who live in cultures that have sanctions against the expression of pain tend to express less pain. Sanctions against showing pain are probably also the reason why _____ express less pain than women do.

C. Theories of Pain

Pain is a complex phenomenon that is not completely understood, giving rise to several theories of pain. The two leading models of pain are the _____ theory, which hypothesizes the existence of a specific pain pathway that makes the experience of pain virtually equal to the amount of tissue damage or injury. The second and generally more accepted theory is the _____ _____ theory proposed by Ronald Melzack and Peter Wall. This theory hypothesizes that a gating mechanism exists in the _____ _____, specifically in the structure called the _____ _____ of the dorsal horns of the spinal cord. This modulation can change pain perception, as can brain-level alterations from a hypothesized _____ _____ trigger. This theory includes explanations of both physiological and psychological modulations of the pain experience. Melzack has proposed an extension to the gate control theory that puts an even stronger emphasis on the brain's role in pain perception, an extension called _____ theory.

III. The Measurement of Pain

A number of techniques have been used to measure laboratory and clinical pain, and these fall into three main categories: self-reports, behavioral assessments, and physiological measures.

A. Self-Reports

Self-report measures of pain include rating scales, standardized pain inventories, and standardized personality inventories. With rating scales, patients are asked to rate the intensity of their pain on a scale—for example, from 1 to 100. Melzack developed an inventory that categorizes pain into sensory, affective, and evaluative dimensions. This inventory is called the _____ Pain Inventory. Another attempt to assess pain is the Multidimensional Pain Inventory. Standardized psychological tests, such as the

_____ _____ _____ _____ (MMPI), have also been used to assess pain and have some ability to differentiate among types of pain patients.

B. Behavioral Assessment

Health psychologists have used observation of _____ to assess pain, looking at the ways that people in pain communicate that pain to others. In addition to trained observers, significant others, such as spouses or other family, can also rate pain behaviors. This method can be especially useful to evaluate the pain of _____ or older people who cannot express their pain in language.

C. Physiological Measures

Several physiological variables have the potential to measure pain, including muscle tension and autonomic indices. Muscle tension as measured by

_____ (EMG) has an inconsistent relationship with perceived pain severity, but autonomic indices such as skin temperature show some promise.

IV. Pain Syndromes

Pain can be classified according to location or syndrome.

A. Headache Pain

Headaches are the most frequent pain syndrome in the United States. The most common varieties are migraine, tension, and cluster headaches. _____ headaches bring about loss of appetite, nausea, vomiting, and increased sensitivity to light. Those headaches caused by contractions of the muscles of the neck, shoulders, scalp, and face are _____ headaches. Headaches that produce intense pain localized in one side of the head and occur frequently over a period of days are _____ headaches.

B. Low Back Pain

Another common pain syndrome is low back pain, which has many causes. The most common cause of low back pain is _____, but psychological factors may also be involved. For example, people with low back pain may be exempt from unpleasant tasks, which can perpetuate their pain behaviors and _____ their recovery. Only about _____% of people with low back pain have an identifiable cause for their pain.

C. Arthritis Pain

A variety of arthritic pains exist, and many involve inflammation of the joints. Perhaps the most frequent cause of arthritic pain is an autoimmune disorder called _____ _____, which is characterized by a dull ache within or around a joint. A progressive inflammation of the joints that is characterized by a dull ache in the joint area and tends to affect older people is called _____.

D. Cancer Pain

Cancer pain is present in about two thirds of all cancer cases. Cancer pain may be caused by either the cancer itself or by the _____ of the cancer.

E. Phantom Limb Pain

Amputees nearly always continue to feel some sensation in the missing body part, and the feeling is frequently painful. This experience of chronic pain in an amputated part of the body is known as _____ _____ _____.

V. Managing Pain

Managing either acute or chronic pain presents challenges, but _____ pain is more difficult because it has no identifiable cause.

A. Medical Approaches to Managing Pain

Medical treatments can manage pain, but pain patients may not receive adequate medication because medical personnel tend to _____ patients' pain. The most common treatment for acute pain is _____ drugs. These drugs are usually either of the aspirin type or the opiate type. Aspirin is one of the _____

_____-_____ drugs (NSAIDs). Along with ibuprofen and naproxen sodium, these drugs are useful in managing minor pain, but more powerful analgesic effects can be obtained from _____ drugs. The fear that this drug will cause addiction and other drug-related problems prevents many physicians from prescribing it.

The most drastic form of treatment for chronic pain is surgery either to repair damage or to prevent nerves from relaying pain messages. Unfortunately, surgery is often unsuccessful in alleviating _____ pain and often produces additional unwanted effects.

B. Behavioral Interventions for Managing Pain

Behavioral interventions for managing pain include relaxation training, behavior modification, cognitive therapy, and cognitive behavioral therapy. Progressive _____ relaxation involves learning to relax the entire body, one muscle group at a time, and to breathe deeply and exhale slowly. A National Institute of Health Technology panel's evaluation for pain treatments gave relaxation training its _____ rating. _____ _____ techniques are based on the principles of operant conditioning and are used by health psychologists to help people cope with stress and pain. People in pain may continue their pain behaviors because they receive _____ such as attention, sympathy, financial compensation, relief from work, and other rewards. The goal of behavior modification is to _____ the pain patient's environment to discontinue reinforcement for pain behaviors.

Cognitive therapy assumes that a change in the interpretation of an event can change people's emotional and physiological reaction to that event. When pain patients _____ differently about their pain experiences, the experience may change. Cognitive _____ therapy aims to develop beliefs, thoughts, and skills to make positive changes in behavior. Dennis Turk and Donald Meichenbaum have developed a cognitive behavioral program for pain management called_____ _____, which involves the cognitive stage of _____ and the behavioral stages of acquisition and rehearsal of _____ and follow-through.

Multiple Choice Questions

_____ 1. Individuals with chronic pain insensitivity demonstrate that
   a. lack of pain sensation allows people to live longer lives.
   b. a life without pain is undesirable.
   c. a life without pain increases happiness.
   d. lack of pain sensation is a disadvantage for adults but an advantage for children.

_____ 2. The _____ system permits people to interpret certain sensory information as pain.
   a. muscular
   b. skeletal
   c. endocrine
   d. somatosensory

_____ 3. Sensory impulses are conveyed directly to the spinal cord by
   a. primary afferents.
   b. secondary afferents.
   c. the peripheral nervous system.
   d. motor neurons.

_____ 4. The dorsal horns are located in the
   a. midbrain.
   b. myelin.
   c. spinal cord.
   d. brain stem.

_____ 5. The substantia gelatinosa
   a. connects afferent neurons to efferent neurons.
   b. receives information from the efferent system.
   c. is capable of modulating sensory input.
   d. none of the above.

_____ 6. Alice has just smashed her finger with a hammer. She experiences _____ pain.
   a. chronic
   b. chronic intractable
   c. prechronic
   d. acute

_____ 7. Which of these is a distinction between chronic and acute pain?
   a. Chronic pain is usually adaptive; acute pain is not.
   b. Acute pain is physical; chronic pain is psychological.
   c. Chronic pain is often prolonged by environmental reinforcers; acute pain needs no such reinforcement.
   d. Chronic pain warns us to avoid further injury; acute pain has no such warning ability.

_____ 8. After studying wounded soldiers and wounded civilians, Henry Beecher concluded that
   a. civilians experienced less pain than soldiers.
   b. pain is both psychological and physical.
   c. the experience of pain is directly proportional with the level of tissue damage.
   d. pain is almost totally physical.

_____ 9. John Bonica believed that chronic pain results from tissue damage plus
   a. a vulnerability to stress.
   b. number of stressful life events.
   c. a hostile attitude toward people.
   d. previous experiences of being rewarded for pain behaviors.

_____ 10. What theory of pain assumes that a person's experience of pain is virtually equal to the degree of tissue damage?
   a. specificity theory
   b. sensory decision theory
   c. the gate control theory
   d. all of the above

_____ 11. The gate control theory of pain was proposed by
   a. Bonica.
   b. Lazarus.
   c. Melzack and Wall.
   d. Turk and Meichenbaum.

_____ 12. The gate control theory of pain assumes that
   a. the spinal cord modulates the input of sensory information.
   b. the cerebellum is mostly responsible for the sensation of pain.
   c. individual perception is mostly responsible for the feeling of pain.
   d. classical conditioning experiences are largely responsible for the sensation of pain.

_____ 13. Which of the following is NOT a method that health psychologists use to measure pain?
   a. behavioral observation
   b. self-reports
   c. the Social Readjustment Rating Scale
   d. physiological measures

_____ 14. Asking physicians to estimate their patients' pain is not a valid measurement because
   a. physicians' estimates correlate with patients' estimates.
   b. physicians rely on behaviors that signal pain, which are not valid measures of pain.
   c. physicians overestimate patients' pain.
   d. physicians underestimate patients' pain.

_____ 15. The most commonly used measurement of pain is the
   a. Minnesota Multiphasic Personality Inventory.
   b. McGill Pain Questionnaire.
   c. Beck Depression Inventory.
   d. observational method.

_____ 16. In general, judgments of observers trained to identify pain behaviors are
   a. unreliable.
   b. moderately reliable.
   c. somewhat reliable but have no validity.
   d. both reliable and valid.

_____ 17. In the United States, more people experience what type of pain than any other?
   a. low back pain
   b. headache
   c. acute
   d. chronic recurrent

_____ 18. Cassandra experiences recurrent pain that is accompanied by sensitivity to light, loss of appetite, and nausea. The most likely diagnosis is
   a. tension headaches.
   b. migraine headaches.
   c. low back pain.
   d. phantom limb pain.

_____ 19. Preston is a 45-year-old librarian who has never experienced a migraine headache. His chances of a first migraine are
   a. very low.
   b. about one in five.
   c. about 50/50.
   d. very high.

_____ 20. Rheumatoid arthritis, unlike osteoarthritis,
   a. is an autoimmune disorder.
   b. occurs only in elderly people.
   c. often develops into chronic pain.
   d. all of the above.

_____ 21. Cancer patients with this type of cancer are least likely to suffer severe pain.
   a. bone cancer
   b. cervical cancer
   c. metastatic cancer
   d. leukemia

_____ 22. Phantom limb pain
   a. is the same as stump pain.
   b. does not occur in women who have had a breast removed.
   c. increases in frequency as time goes by.
   d. none of the above.

_____ 23. Treatment for _____ pain is easier than treatment for _____.
   a. severe . . . minor
   b. chronic . . . acute
   c. acute . . . chronic
   d. daily . . . intermittent

_____ 24. Opiate drugs
   a. are not effective analgesics.
   b. can produce dependence.
   c. do not produce tolerance.
   d. all of the above.

_____ 25. What type of medication includes aspirin and ibuprofen?
   a. nonsteroidal anti-inflammatory drugs
   b. acetaminophens
   c. opiate drugs
   d. none of the above

_____ 26. Tyler has suffered low back pain for several years and tried many treatments. He is now considering _____, which is usually the last resort for pain treatment.
   a. opiate drugs
   b. NSAIDs
   c. TENS
   d. surgery

_____ 27. How great is the risk of addiction for patients who have received opiate drugs while in the hospital?
   a. About 50% of patients who receive opiates become addicted.
   b. Addiction is a problem for people who receive these drugs for acute pain, but people with chronic pain rarely develop an addiction.
   c. About 70% of patients who receive opiate develop a dependence, but only about 15% develop a tolerance.
   d. Only about 1% of people who receive opiate drugs in the hospital develop an addiction.

_____ 28. What management strategy relies heavily on operant conditioning principles?
   a. biofeedback
   b. cognitive therapy
   c. behavior modification
   d. relaxation training

_____ 29. Marcie's husband is constantly complaining about pain in his lower back. He also walks with a limp and moans audibly when he is near Marcie. To help her husband, Marcie should
    a. ignore her husband's complaints, limps, and moans.
    b. seek medical treatment for her husband.
    c. give her husband daily back massages.
    d. do all the heavy lifting in her house.

_____ 30. The management strategy that emphasizes changing the way people think about their pain is
    a. cognitive therapy.
    b. behavior modification.
    c. biofeedback.
    d. hypnosis.

_____ 31. Although drug treatments may be very effective for managing acute pain, _____ is a better choice for chronic pain.
    a. hypnosis
    b. cognitive behavioral therapy
    c. opiates
    d. biofeedback

Key Terms

Define each of the following:

A-beta fibers —

acute pain —

analgesic drugs —

behavior modification —

C fibers —

chronic pain —

gate control theory —

nociceptors —

opiate drugs —

periaqueductal gray —

phantom limb pain —

positive reinforcer —

somatosensory system —

substantia gelatinosa —

tolerance —

Matching

Match the following:

1. nociceptors	a. endogenous opiate
2. substantia gelatinosa	b. in the parietal lobe of the cerebral cortex
3. primary afferents	c. tolerance and dependence
4. somatosensory cortex	d. most frequent measurement of pain
5. periaqueductal gray	e. neurons with receptors in the sense organs
6. opiate drugs	f. midbrain structure capable of modulating pain
7. endorphin	g. neurons capable of sensing pain.
8. Melzack and Wall	h. most common pain syndrome
9. McGill Pain Questionnaire	i. gate control theory
10. headache	j. laminae 1 and 2 in the dorsal horns of the spinal cord

1. _____ 2. _____ 3. _____ 4. _____ 5. _____

6. _____ 7. _____ 8. _____ 9. _____ 10. _____

Opening and Closing the Gate

Fill in the missing information to represent the gate control mechanism for conditions that promote and for conditions that decrease pain perception.

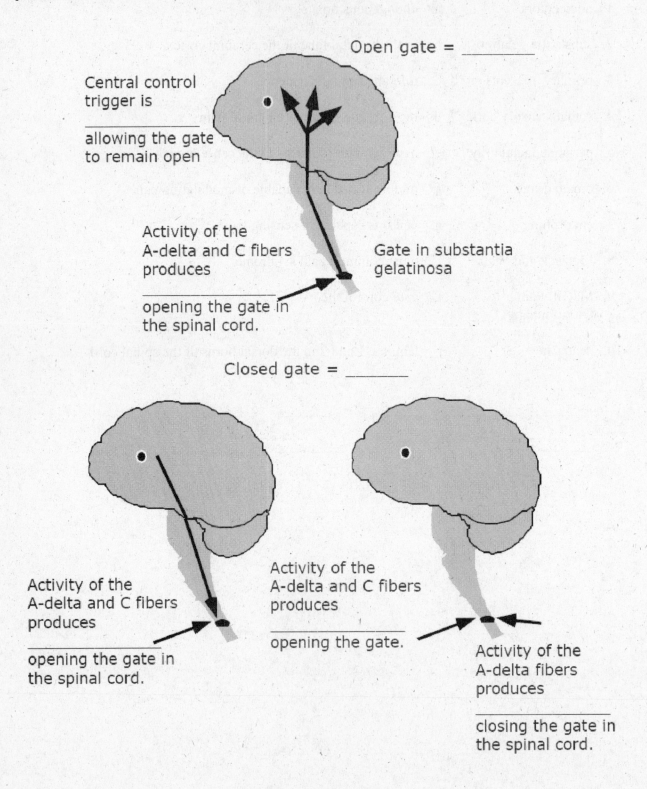

Open gate = _____

Central control trigger is

_____ allowing the gate to remain open

Activity of the A-delta and C fibers produces

_____ opening the gate in the spinal cord.

Gate in substantia gelatinosa

Closed gate = _____

Activity of the A-delta and C fibers produces

_____ opening the gate in the spinal cord.

Activity of the A-delta and C fibers produces

_____ opening the gate.

Activity of the A-delta fibers produces

_____ closing the gate in the spinal cord.

Essay Questions

1. Bryan cut his ankle. What could decrease his experience of the pain resulting from the cut?

2. Evaluate the statement, "Context is more important than personality in the experience of pain."

3. Which behavioral techniques are effective for coping with pain?

Let's Get Personal— Charting Your Pain

Except people with chronic pain insensitivity, everyone experiences pain. For most people, acute pain is a common but not a serious event. For others, chronic pain is part of their lives every day. To help understand your pain, keep a pain diary for at least a week and preferably for longer.

Record the following information, and after keeping a record of your pain experience for at least a week, decide what role pain plays in your life

Day—

Time of day—

Source of the pain—

Severity of the pain—

Barely   Worst Pain
Painful   Imaginable

1   2   3   4   5   6   7   8   9   10

I coped with the pain by

Other people did/did not know that I was in pain because I

Those people who knew I was in pain reacted by

This pain caused me to make the following changes in my daily routine

Answers

Fill in the Rest of the Story

I.   brain
I.A.   somatosensory; afferent; nociceptors; A-beta; myelin; C
I.B.   spinal cord; transmission; laminae; substantia gelatinosa
I.C.   thalamus; parietal
I.D.   endorphin; proinflammatory cytokines
I.E.   periaqueductal gray; nucleus raphé magnus
II.A.   emotional; acute; Chronic; prechronic
II.B.   cultural; men
II.C.   specificity; gate control; spinal cord, substantia gelatinosa; central control; neuromatrix
III.A. McGill; Minnesota Multiphasic Personality Inventory
III.B. behavior; children
III.C. electromyography
IV.A.   Migraine; tension; cluster
IV.B.   injury; prevent (slow); 20
IV.C.   rheumatoid arthritis; osteoarthritis
IV.D.   treatment
IV.E   phantom limb pain
V.   chronic
V.A.   underestimate; analgesic; nonsteroidal anti-inflammatory; opiate; chronic
V.B.   muscle; highest; Behavior modification; reinforcement (rewards); change (alter); think; behavioral; pain inoculation; reconceptualization; skills

Multiple Choice Answers

1. b	9. d	17. b	25. a
2. d	10. a	18. b	26. d
3. a	11. c	19. a	27. d
4. c	12. a	20. a	28. c
5. c	13. c	21. d	29. a
6. d	14. d	22. d	30. a
7. c	15. b	23. c	31. b
8. b	16. d	24. b	

Matching

1. g	2. j	3. e	4. b	5. f
6. c	7. a	8. i	9. d	10. h

Good points to include in your essay answers:

1. A. If Bryan has a congenital insensitivity to pain, then the cut did not hurt, but this situations very unlikely.
   B. Bryan's pain would probably be decreased if
      1. He was involved with some other distracting activity when the cut occurred.
      2. He was not looking at his ankle when the injury occurred.
      3. He did not look at his ankle after the cut so that he did not see the extent of his injury.
      4. He pressed tightly on the cut, stimulating other neurons in addition to the ones arrying pain messages and partially blocking the pain.
      5. He experienced some other injury in another part of his body, producing another type nd location of pain.
      6. He believed that men should not be bothered by minor injuries or that he was the type f man who should not feel pain by such an injury.

2. A. Personality is not a very good predictor of reactions to pain.
      1. No evidence supports the existence of a pain-prone personality.
      2. No evidence supports the existence of a pain-resistant personality.
   B. Situational factors are more important than personality in the experience of pain. Pain ensitivity and the expression of pain behaviors show large cultural variations.
      1. Cultural expectations influence women's behavior during childbirth.
      2. Ethnic background influences the expression of pain behaviors.
      3. Ethnic background influences the treatment that people receive when they are in ain, with African Americans and Hispanic Americans receiving less attention and reatment for their complaints of pain.
      4. Gender differences in the expression of pain may also be attributable to gender roles nd differing expectation for women and men.

3. A. Each of the medical treatments for pain has both advantages and disadvantages.
   B. Analgesic drug treatments are common.
      1. Opiate drugs are very successful in relieving severe pain, but they produce tolerance nd dependence, creating the potential for abuse and making these drugs less suitable or the management of chronic than for acute pain.
      2. Nonsteroidal anti-inflammatory drugs (NSAIDs) and other over-the-counter nalgesics can be effective for acute pain and sometimes for chronic pain, but they are ot as effective as opiates.
   C. Surgery is less common than analgesic drugs and less successful.
      1. Severing nerves can prevent pain messages from reaching the brain, but all surgery arries hazards.
      2. Any effect, including unpleasant ones, will be permanent.
      3. Surgery usually does not produce relief from chronic pain.

CHAPTER 8
Considering Alternative Approaches

Learning Objectives

After studying Chapter 8, you should be able to

1. Explain the differences between conventional and alternative medicine.
2. Discuss alternative medical systems.
3. Analyze the similarities and differences among the practices and products used in alternative medicine.
4. Provide a rationale for mind-body medicine.
5. Describe the most commonly used mind-body techniques.
6. Discuss who uses alternative medicine and the reasons for that decision.
7. Evaluate the evidence for the most effective alternative treatments and identify the conditions for which each is effective.
8. Describe the limitations of alternative treatments.
9. Identify the advantages and the barriers to the development of integrative medicine.

Fill in the Rest of the Story

I. Alternative Medical Systems

Conventional medicine is a term applied to treatments that arose within Western culture. Other cultures hold different views of health and _____ that lead to different medical treatments. When people in Western cultures use these treatments rather than conventional treatments, they are using _____ medicine. When they combine these alternative treatments with conventional ones, the term _____ medicine applies. These terms are often combined into complementary and alternative medicine or _____. The U.S. National Center for Complementary and Alternative Medicine is an agency created to prompt evaluation of alternative treatments.

A. Traditional Chinese Medicine

Traditional _____ medicine (TCM) originated in China over 2,000 years ago. This system is based on the concept that a vital force called _____ (or *chi*) flows through the body. If the flow is blocked or becomes stagnant, illness can occur. Attaining a balance between the two opposing energy forces of _____ and _____ is essential for maintaining health. TCM practitioners use acupuncture and _____, massage called _____ _____, herbal preparations, the energy-channeling exercises of qi gong and _____ _____.

B. Ayurvedic Medicine

Ayurvedic medicine, or _____, originated in India over 2,000 years ago. Its goal is to integrate and _____ the body, soul, and mind, which is accomplished through changes in diet and exercise, which includes _____, massage, and preparations made with oils, minerals, and spices.

C. Naturopathy

The system of _____ arose in 19th century Europe and holds the view that bodies have the power to maintain and return to a state of health through a healthy_____, fresh air, exercise, and exposure to _____.

D. Homeopathy

_____ arose in the 1700s in Germany, based on the principle that "like cures _____"; that is, substances have curative power when they produce symptoms that are similar to those of the disease. _____ is the notion that systematically diluting a substance and shaking it vigorously after each dilution makes the mixture more rather than less potent, which is the basis of homeopathic _____.

II. Alternative Practices and Products

Alternative practices and products include chiropractic treatments, massage, energy healing, diets, and dietary supplements.

A. Chiropractic Treatment

Chiropractic was founded in 1895 by Daniel David Palmer, who believed that manipulation of the _____ was the key to curing and preventing disease. Chiropractic practitioners receive doctoral degrees and perform _____ to the spine and joints to correct misalignments. The fight for acceptance has been successful; about _____% of people in the United States use chiropractic care each year.

B. Massage

Massage manipulates _____ _____ to produce health benefits and allows the body to heal itself. Several different types of massage exist, including _____ massage, acupressure (and its Japanese counterpart Shiatsu), tui na, and Ayurvedic massage.

C. Energy Healing

The view that energy can heal the body or that the body contains vital, healing energy is common to many alternative systems. Energy healing techniques seek to channel the body's healing energy and include _____ _____ exercises from traditional Chinese medicine and _____, a massage technique from Japan. The technique of _____ _____ is intended to direct the energy fields of the body, but without actually touching the person.

D. Diets

Many people follow specialized _____ oriented to weight loss or lowering

cholesterol levels, such as the _____, Ornish, or Zone diets; other diets have the

goal of improving health, such as _____ and macrobiotic diets.

E. Dietary Supplements

Dietary supplements include _____ and minerals, which people use to preserve

health and promote wellness, but some supplements are used as cures. In addition,

supplements include _____ _____, which are biologically active

components of diet, such as fish oil, chocolate, and cranberries.

III. Mind—Body Medicine

Mind–body medicine is the term applied to a variety of techniques that are based on the

notion that the _____, mind, body, and _____ interact in complex ways and that

emotional, mental, social, and behavioral factors exert important effects on health

A. Meditation and Yoga

Meditative techniques and yoga allow people to relax. _____ _____

directs people to focus on a single thought or sound to achieve relaxation, whereas

_____ meditation encourages practitioners to focus on the moment, becoming

mindful of the details of their current experience. Guided imagery asks patients to imagine

a _____ scene and to concentrate on that image throughout a stressful

or painful situation. _____ uses physical postures, breathing, and meditation, with

the goal of balancing body, mind, and spirit.

B. Qi Gong and Tai Chi

The movement-based practices of _____ _____ and _____ _____ originated in traditional Chinese medicine. Qi gong and tai chi involve postures and movements that are intended to balance the body's energy and restore health.

C. Biofeedback

Biofeedback is the process of providing feedback information about the status of _____ systems, which permits people to alter physiological responses that could not have been voluntarily controlled without the feedback. The two biofeedback procedures most frequently used in clinical practice are the

_____ (EMG), which measures electrical discharge in muscle fibers, and _____ biofeedback, which uses a thermister to measure skin temperature.

D. Hypnotic Treatment

Hypnotic procedures are ancient, but the modern form can be traced to _____. Authorities currently disagree concerning the precise nature of hypnosis; some argue that hypnosis is an _____ state of consciousness, but others view hypnosis as a generalized trait. Those who see it as an altered state of consciousness believe that an _____ is necessary to achieve the state, but all agree that it includes focused attention and that all hypnosis is _____-

_____.

IV. Who Uses Complementary and Alternative Medicine?

CAM is growing in popularity in the United States and in other industrialized countries. Excluding those who used prayers for health, 36% of people surveyed in the U.S. used some form of alternative medicine within a year of the survey. Including those who used prayer,

_____% used some type of alternative medicine. Rather than substituting one or more of the alternative approaches, a majority of people added an alternative treatment to their conventional treatment. That is, most people use such techniques as _____ and not _____ medicine.

A. Culture, Ethnicity, and Gender

People in Australia and some _____ countries are more likely to use CAM than people in the United States. The typical person who uses CAM in the United States is well-educated, in a high income group, and of _____-_____ ethnicity.

B. Motivations for Seeking Alternative Treatment

People who seek alternative treatment have a worldview that is consistent with such an approach; these people are more likely to accept the _____ view than the biomedical view of disease. In addition, people whose medical condition has not responded to _____ treatment are more likely to seek alternative treatment.

V. How Effective Are Alternative Treatments?

For alternative treatments to be accepted by conventional medicine, _____ evidence must confirm their effectiveness, but few randomized, _____ trials have been conducted on CAM treatments. However, evidence for the effectiveness of CAM is growing.

A. Alternative Treatments for Anxiety, Stress, and Depression

Transcendental and mindfulness _____ are effective in managing anxiety, and _____-based stress reduction is a good approach for managing _____. The movement-based practices of _____ _____ and tai chi are also effective in helping to manage stress. Acupuncture and _____ show some promise of reducing depression, and the herbal remedy _____-_____ _____

has also been found to reduce depression.

B. Alternative Treatments for Pain

Guided imagery seems to be an effective intervention in helping people manage several

types of _____. Techniques from traditional Chinese medicine have been successful

in pain management. Qi gong and _____ _____ show promise in such chronic

pain problems as headache and fibromyalgia. Acupuncture can be effective for easing low

back pain, but _____ and _____ treatment are also effective for this

pain syndrome. Chiropractic treatment is also effective for neck and musculoskeletal pain.

However, biofeedback is no more effective for managing headache or low back pain than

_____ _____. Hypnosis is effective for a variety of types of pain

but is more effective for _____ pain such as postsurgical and burn pain than for

_____ pain.

C. Alternative Treatments for Other Conditions

Research also indicates that techniques from CAM are effective for a variety of other

conditions. For example, _____ _____ speeds burn healing; hypnosis and

_____ can both help in controlling nausea and vomiting.

_____ biofeedback is effective in managing Raynaud's disease, and the

practice of _____ _____ and tai chi can alter the immune system in beneficial

ways. _____ _____ decreases fear of falling and improves balance and

flexibility in older adults

D. Limitations of Alternative Therapy

The primary limitation for alternative medicine is the _____ of research

on its effectiveness, but the National Center for Complementary and Alternative Medicine is beginning to solve this problem. Individuals with some conditions should avoid some treatments; for example, people with weakened bones should be cautious in seeking _____ or _____ treatment. CAM is also limited in its accessibility: CAM treatment is not available in all locations, and the _____ of treatment may limit who has access because services are often not covered by insurance.

E. Integrative Medicine

The movement toward _____ medicine is an attempt to integrate alternative and conventional treatments to provide improved treatment. Although this integration faces challenges, some _____ clinics and _____ treatment programs offer integrative medicine.

Multiple Choice Questions

_____ 1. A treatment is considered to be alternative medicine when
    a. that treatment is ineffective.
    b. that treatment produces effects no larger than the placebo effect.
    c. that treatment is not accepted within conventional medicine.
    d. the alternative to the treatment is death.

_____ 2. The difference between complementary and alternative medicine
    a. is a matter of acceptance by the medical community.
    b. depends on whether a person uses the treatment rather than conventional treatment or combined with conventional treatment.
    c. depends on how many people use a treatment—more people use alternative and complementary treatments.
    d. depends on who is defining the two fields because no standard definitions exist.

_____ 3. Traditional Chinese medicine holds that a vital force flows through the body. That force is called _____, which flows through a system of _____.
    a. yang . . . ducts
    b. blood . . . veins
    c. energy . . . reservoirs
    d. qi . . . meridians

_____ 4. Ayurvedic medicine strives to bring a balance
   a. among body, mind, and spirit.
   b. among family members.
   c. between the energies derived from the sun and the earth.
   d. between the forces of yin and yang.

_____ 5. All alternative medical systems
   a. have become well accepted among medical practitioners in the United States and Europe.
   b. conceptualize health as holistic, considering psychological as well as physical factors in health and disease.
   c. have demonstrated a clear physical basis for their practices and products.
   d. view the person as passive and the universe as active.

_____ 6. Most people who use prayer for health improvements report that they find prayer helpful in this respect. Research indicates that
   a. people who attend religious services on a daily basis have more heart attacks than people who do not attend religious services.
   b. people's health improves when these people know that they are the recipients of prayers but not when they are unaware of the prayers.
   c. whether or not prayers are beneficial depends on the age of the targets, with older people receiving more benefits from prayers than younger people.
   d. people who attend religious services have a high level of interpersonal hostility and experience more social isolation than those who do not.

_____ 7. Manipulation of soft tissue is the definition of _____, and _____ is defined as manipulation of the spine to achieve therapeutic benefits.
   a. TENS . . . massage
   b. massage . . . chiropractic treatment
   c. acupuncture . . . acupressure
   d. qi gong . . . acupuncture

_____ 8. What relaxation technique involves patients focusing nonjudgmentally on any thoughts or sensations that occur to them in order to gain insight into how they see the world?
   a. guided imagery
   b. mindfulness meditation
   c. meditative relaxation
   d. rational emotive therapy

_____ 9. Qi gong is
   a. a Japanese form of acupuncture.
   b. a type of spinal manipulation that has therapeutic effects.
   c. a series of movements that has therapeutic benefits.
   d. a type of exercise that increases strength and flexibility but carries risks for all but those in good physical condition.

_____10. The technique whereby patients learn to control their biological processes such as heart rate or skin temperature is known as
   a. biofeedback.
   b. mindfulness mediation.
   c. meditative relaxation.
   d. guided imagery.

_____11. Health psychologists generally regard the main benefit of hypnotic treatment to be its ability to help people
   a. stop smoking.
   b. cure insomnia.
   c. comply with medical advice.
   d. manage pain.

_____12. How popular is CAM in the United States?
   a. Quite popular—over one third of the people in the United States use some form of CAM.
   b. Very popular—over 90% of the people in the United States use some form of CAM.
   c. Not very popular—only about 15% of people in the United States use some form of CAM.
   d. CAM is popular among immigrants to the United States and less educated people but not among college graduates.

_____13. Relaxation training, including forms of meditation, has been most successful in
   a. treating mental disorders rather than physical diseases.
   b. treating ulcers and other psychosomatic disorders.
   c. managing stress and anxiety.
   d. helping children and adolescents manage school-related problems.

_____14. As a treatment for pain, acupuncture
   a. is more effective for some people than for others.
   b. is no more effective than a placebo.
   c. cannot produce analgesia in animals.
   d. is effective among Chinese but not Europeans.

_____15. What CAM treatments have demonstrated effectiveness in managing low back pain?
   a. chiropractic treatment
   b. acupuncture
   c. massage
   d. all of the above

_____16.   The benefits of biofeedback
  a.   come mainly from relaxation rather than from the process of controlling physiological responses.
  b.   are restricted to well-educated adults.
  c.   include lowering high blood pressure into the normal range for more than 50% of those who receive cardiac biofeedback.
  d.   are greater than hypnosis for managing low back pain.

_____17.   What patients are most likely to benefit from hypnotic treatment when it is used to relieve pain?
  a.   children
  b.   people low in suggestibility
  c.   people high in suggestibility
  d.   elderly men

_____18.   Hypnosis is more effective in controlling _____ pain than _____ pain.
  a.   burn . . . postsurgical
  b.   chronic . . . headache
  c.   acute . . . chronic
  d.   arthritis . . . muscular

_____19.   The movement-based therapies of qi gong and tai chi have benefits
  a.   for older people but not for younger ones.
  b.   that include relieving pain and developing better sensory abilities.
  c.   that include relaxation, increases in muscle strength, and improved balance.
  d.   that can be attributed to a placebo response.

_____20.   One of the limitations on CAM comes from
  a.   limitations on access to such treatments due to the costs.
  b.   limitations on the effectiveness of any CAM therapy to manage pain.
  c.   limitations on the effectiveness of any CAM therapy to improve mood or depression.
  d.   all of the above.

_____21.   Integrative medicine
  a.   describes the combination of drugs and surgery to treat chronic pain.
  b.   is an attempt to integrate treatment so that the ethnic disparities in health care disappear.
  c.   is an attempt to combine conventional and alternative medicine to benefit patient treatment.
  d.   has been proposed but not yet attempted.

Key Terms

Define each of the following:

acupuncture —

alternative medicine —

Ayurveda —

biofeedback —

complementary medicine —

induction —

integrative medicine —

naturopathy —

Matching

Match the following:

1. naturopathy
2. integrative medicine
3. Atkins, Ornish, Zone, and Pritikin
4. chiropractic treatment
5. EMG
6. Ayurveda
7. qi gong and tai chi
8. guided imagery
9. basis of mind-body medicine
10. suggestibility

a. brain, mind, and body interact in complex ways

b. type of relaxation training

c. manipulation of the spine

d. allows people to be hypnotized

e. medical system that promotes healthy diet, fresh air, and exercise as routes to healing

f. movement-based therapies

g. combination of alternative and conventional medicine

h. system of medicine that arose in ancient India

i. types of diets

j. type of biofeedback

1. _____ 2. _____ 3. _____ 4. _____ 5. _____

6. _____ 7. _____ 8. _____ 9. _____ 10. _____

Essay Questions

1. Evaluate the statement, "Alternative medicine has become widely accepted in the United States."

2. Discuss the effectiveness of alternative treatments.

Let's Get Personal—

Attitudes about alternative approaches to health care vary, but college students tend to be more receptive to such treatments than many other people. Most college students have not received alternative treatment. You probably have an opinion of your likelihood of seeking some alternative treatment, but that overall opinion may be changed by an analysis of your health concerns and the evidence about the effectiveness and availability of such treatment.

Think of at least two problems or concerns for which you receive treatment or would profit from receiving treatment. Such problems may include stress, anxiety, weight concerns, sleep problems, headaches, low back pain, or other conditions. Complete the exercise by evaluating the effectiveness, risks, availability and costs of various alternative treatments.

Tables 8.3-8.5 in the text include information that will help you evaluate the effectiveness of various treatments, but you may consult other sources as well. Remember that information from the Internet requires your critical evaluation. For example, most .com websites attempt to sell services or products, so their claims require careful evaluation independent of the claims on the website. Other considerations include the potential risks and dangers of the alternative treatment and the availability and cost of such interventions.

When you have gathered this information and filled out the form, you will have a summary of the positive and negative points of this treatment for your problem. Make an overall rating of the alternative treatments you explored. Perhaps you will discover an alternative or complementary treatment you would not have considered.

Problem #1 _____

	Evidence for Effectiveness Lacking . . . . Strong	Risks	Availability/ Cost	Rating
Chiropractic				
Massage				
Diets				
Dietary Supplements				
Meditation				
Yoga				
Tai Chi/ Qi Gong				
Biofeedback				
Hypnosis				
Homeopathic Remedies				

Problem #2 _____

	Evidence for Effectiveness Lacking . . . . Strong	Risks	Availability/ Cost	Rating
Chiropractic				
Massage				
Diets				
Dietary Supplements				
Meditation				
Yoga				
Tai Chi/ Qi Gong				
Biofeedback				
Hypnosis				
Homeopathic Remedies				

Answers

Fill in the Rest of the Story

I.   disease (illness); alternative; complementary; CAM
I.A.   Chinese; qi; yin; yang; acupressure; tui na; tai chi
I.B.   Ayurveda; balance; yoga
I.C.   naturopathy; diet; sunlight
I.D.   Homeopathy; like; Potentization; remedies
II.A.   spine; adjustments; 8
II.B.   soft tissue; Swedish
II.C.   qi gong; Reiki; Therapeutic Touch
II.D.   diets; Atkins; vegetarian
II.E.   vitamins; functional foods
III.   brain; behavior
III.A. Transcendental meditation; mindfulness; pleasant; Yoga
III.B. qi gong; tai chi
III.C. physiological (biological); electromyograph; temperature (thermal)
III.D. Mesmer; altered; induction; self-hypnosis
IV.   63; complementary; alternative
IV.A.   European; European-American
IV.B.   biopsychosocial; conventional
V.   research; controlled
V.A.   meditation; mindfulness; stress; qi gong; yoga; Saint-John's wort
V.B.   stress; tai chi; massage; chiropractic; relaxation training; acute; chronic
V.C.   aloe vera; acupuncture; Thermal; qi gong; Tai chi
V.D.   lack; massage; chiropractic; cost
V.E.   integrative; pain; cancer

Multiple Choice

1. c	6. b	11. d	16. a
2. b	7. b	12. a	17. c
3. d	8. b	13. c	18. c
4. a	9. c	14. a	19. c
5. b	10. a	15. d	20. a
			21. c

Matching

1. e	2. g	3. i	4. c	5. j
6. h	7. f	8. b	9. a	10. d

Good points to include in your essay answers:

1. A. In some sense, this statement is true.
        1. Sixty-three percent of people in the United States say that they have used some form of alternative medicine within the past year (36% when excluding the use of prayer).
        2. Use of natural and herbal products, chiropractic treatment, massage therapy, yoga, and meditation are becoming increasingly common.
    B. In some sense, the statement is not true.
        1. Most of the people who use alternative medicine combine these techniques with conventional medicine.
        2. Only 28% of people who use alternative medicine do so because they believe conventional medicine will not help them.
        3. A more accurate statement would be that complementary (rather than alternative) medicine is increasingly popular.

2. A. Research evidence from high-quality studies on the effectiveness of alternative treatments is not plentiful, but studies are beginning to show that alternative treatments are effective for a variety of conditions.
    B. Meditation procedures include transcendental meditation, mindfulness meditation, and guided imagery.
        1. Transcendental and mindfulness meditation are effective for managing anxiety, mood disorders, and depression.
        2. Mindfulness meditation has been used successfully for stress-related problems.
        3. Guided imagery has some effectiveness in the control of pain related to pregnancy and childbirth, headache pain, and postoperative pain.
    C. Research has demonstrated the effectiveness of qi gong and tai chi for several conditions.
        1. Qi gong is useful in managing several types of chronic pain, including fibromyalgia.
        2. Tai chi is a promising treatment for chronic headaches.
    D. Acupuncture is effective for several pain syndromes, including low back pain, neck pain, and osteoarthritis of the knee.
    E. Chiropractic treatment is effective for back, neck, and musculoskeletal pain.
    F. Hypnotic treatment has been shown to be effective for many types of pain.
        1. These types of pain include pain associated with cancer, dental treatment, burns, headache, low back problems, and childbirth.
        2. Hypnosis is more effective than a placebo for suggestible people but not for others.

CHAPTER 9
Behavioral Factors in Cardiovascular Disease

Learning Objectives

After studying Chapter 9, you should be able to

1. Explain the structure and function of the cardiovascular system.

2. Identify and describe the most common disorders of the cardiovascular system.

3. Distinguish between inherent and acquired risk factors for CVD.

4. Describe how lifestyle relates to the development of cardiovascular disease.

5. Formulate a plan for reducing cardiovascular risk through behavior changes.

Fill in the Rest of the Story

I.   The Cardiovascular System

The cardiovascular system, consisting of the heart and blood vessels, transports

_____ throughout the body, providing a means of delivering oxygen and

nutrients and also removing wastes from cells. Oxygenated blood is carried from the heart by

vessels called _____, and blood that has been released of its oxygen is

returned to the heart by the _____.

A. The Coronary Arteries

Blood is delivered to the myocardium (the _____ muscle) by the

_____ arteries. Any damage to the coronary arteries can be hazardous.

The formation of atheromatous plaque restricts the flow of blood to the myocardium,

resulting in blockage of the arteries called _____. Loss of elasticity or

hardening of the arteries is called _____.

B. Coronary Artery Disease

Coronary artery disease results from the buildup of _____ in the coronary

arteries and may result in damage to the heart, which is _____

_____ _____. One type of coronary heart disease is a restriction of blood flow to the heart, a condition known as _____. This restriction

may produce chest pain and difficulty in breathing and is called _____

_____. Myocardial infarction (often called _____

_____) is a much more serious coronary heart disease.

C. Stroke

When atherosclerosis and arteriosclerosis affect the arteries that deliver blood to the

_____, stroke may occur. A restriction of the _____

supply to the brain, or to part of the brain, results in the death of neurons and the loss of

function performed by those neurons.

D. Blood Pressure

Blood pressure is measured by two numbers: the pressure exerted by ventricular

contractions, called _____ pressure, and the pressure between

contractions, called _____ pressure. High blood pressure, or

_____ may result from several different causes, but the most

common is _____ hypertension, which has no identifiable cause but is a

risk factor for cardiovascular disease. Secondary hypertension is much less common and

results from other disease processes.

II. The Changing Rates of Cardiovascular Disease

Cardiovascular disease is the leading cause of death in the United States, but in recent

years, deaths from heart attack and stroke _____ sharply.

A. Reasons for the Decline in Death Rates

The decline in CVD deaths has been due mostly to two factors: a change to a healthier

_____ of people in the United States and improved medical care for

cardiac patients. Evidence that lifestyle changes play an important role in the decreasing

death rates from CVD is found in research showing a decline in _____ heart

attack. Three lifestyle changes that may have contributed to this decline are: better diet,

increased levels of physical activity, and lower rates of _____.

B. Heart Disease Mortality throughout the World

Countries other than the United States have also experienced lower CVD death rates, but some countries show increases. For example, the rate of CVD in countries that were part of the _____ _____ showed a dramatic increase in heart disease during the 1990s.

III. Risk Factors in Cardiovascular Disease

Much information about risk factors for cardiovascular disease has come from two studies—the _____ Heart Study, begun in 1948 and the 1964 Surgeon General's report on smoking. Results of these and other epidemiological studies have brought the concept of risk factor into popular usage. Risk factors do not prove _____ but simply provide information concerning which conditions are associated with a particular disease.

A. Inherent Risk Factors

Inherent risk factors result from _____ or physical conditions that cannot be changed through modification of lifestyle. One important inherent risk factor for cardiovascular disease is advancing age; for every _____-year increase in age, both women and men double their risk for CVD. A second inherent risk factor is family history; people who have had close relatives die of cardiovascular disease have an increased risk for CVD.

Gender is also an inherent risk; men now have a greater likelihood than women to develop heart disease before age _____ (*see* Figure 9.8). However, this gender difference was quite _____ until about 80 years ago. A fourth inherent risk is _____ background. African Americans have nearly a _____ risk for cardiovascular deaths compared with European Americans. Whether this increased risk for African Americans is inherent or related to social, economic, or behavioral factors remains in question.

B. Physiological Conditions

The best predictor of CVD is _____, or high blood pressure. Another important physiological risk is serum _____, which circulates in the blood in several different forms of lipoprotein. _____-density lipoprotein protects against cardiovascular disease, whereas _____-density lipoprotein contributes to the disease. The *ratio* of total cholesterol to _____- _____ _____ cholesterol seems to be a better predictor of heart disease than total cholesterol. Low-density lipoprotein is difficult to reduce, but eliminating _____ fats (red meats, whole milk, and eggs) from one's diet is effective for many people. Problems in glucose metabolism, including both Type 1 and Type 2 _____ and the metabolic syndrome, raise the risk for heart disease by damaging arteries. Chronic _____ is an immune system response that, even at minor levels, also presents a risk for CVD.

C. Behavioral Factors

The three leading behavioral risk factors for cardiovascular disease are diet, _____, and sedentary lifestyle. Diets high in saturated fat are _____ related to heart disease, whereas those low in saturated fat protect against heart disease. Vitamin E, beta carotene or lycopene, selenium, and riboflavin have been identified as _____ that provide some protection against CVD. Diets high in _____ and _____ offer additional protection against heart disease. Lack of physical _____ is a risk for CVD, but an active lifestyle offers protection. The risks of inactivity begin during _____ and continue throughout the lifespan.

D. Psychosocial Factors

Low educational level and low _____ are both positively related to heart disease. Socioeconomic level is related to a number of factors that are risks for CVD, such as blood pressure and smoking. Indeed, socioeconomic status is related to

_____-_____ mortality.

Having little _____ _____ increases the risk of CVD and

plays a role in its progression. People who are married usually have the support of their

partner, but the _____ of the marital relationship makes a difference,

especially for women.

Stress, anxiety, and _____ are positively related to CVD, but they are

also related to each other, which makes an evaluation of their contribution difficult.

However, the risk from depression applies not only to the development of CVD but also to

its _____.

Since the mid-1980s, evidence for Type A behavior as a coronary risk has become

more complex and less supportive of the original hypothesis. One facet of the Type A

behavior pattern remains of interest as a predictor of heart disease—

_____ hostility. One component of cynical hostility is

_____, which may be the toxic element among the remnants of the

Type A behavior pattern. However, the experience of anger may not be as much of a risk as

its _____. One way that the expression of anger may increase the

risk for CVD is through cardiovascular _____ (CVR), which increases

blood pressure. _____ American men tend to show stronger CVR

than other groups, and they also show higher rates of hypertension. People who

_____ their anger may also experience problems as a result, but the

calm expression of anger may be a healthy way to cope with feelings of anger.

IV. Reducing Cardiovascular Risks

Psychology's main contribution to cardiovascular health is helping people change

_____ that relate to CVD.

A. Before Diagnosis: Preventing First Heart Attacks

People can engage in a number of behaviors that can lower their risk of a heart attack. These include lowering hypertension, reducing cholesterol, and changing psychosocial risk factors. Changing risky behaviors and lifestyles are difficult for several reasons, including the tendency of many people to have an _____ _____.

A difficulty in reducing high blood pressure is that many hypertensive people are _____ of their condition. Adhering to medication for hypertension may be necessary, but weight loss, _____ restriction, exercise, and stress management are several nonpharmacological strategies for reducing hypertension, which may be combined with each other and with drugs to help lower hypertension.

Serum cholesterol is also resistant to changes through behavioral means, but exercise and _____ are two methods that have had some success. Several interventions have been designed to modify cynical hostility and anger, including _____ anger with a calm, slow speech pattern, learning to avoid provocative situations, and using humor.

B. After Diagnosis: Rehabilitating Cardiac Patients

After people have been diagnosed with cardiovascular disease, they typically enter a cardiac _____ program to change their lifestyle and avoid subsequent CVD. Patients recovering from heart disease often experience depression and psychological reactions. _____ survivors have a risk of death 3.5 times greater than do nondepressed patients. Cardiac patients frequently participate in a structured _____ program in which they gradually increase their level of physical activity. Cardiac patients can *reverse* coronary artery damage by massive changes in _____. One such program had the goal of reducing dietary fat, lowering LDL and losing _____.

Multiple Choice Questions

_____ 1. Which one of these persons has the LOWEST risk for heart disease?
  a. a 45-year-old man who openly and loudly expresses anger to other people
  b. a 45-year-old man who suppresses his anger to avoid conflict with others
  c. a 75-year-old European American woman living alone
  d. a 35-year-old European American woman living alone
  e. a 50-year-old African American married man

_____ 2. The circulation of blood
  a. transports carbon dioxide to body cells.
  b. transports oxygen to body cells.
  c. removes carbon dioxide from body cells.
  d. both b and c.

_____ 3. Blood is furnished to the heart by way of
  a. coronary veins.
  b. coronary arteries.
  c. arterioles.
  d. anterior venules.

_____ 4. The technical name for heart attack is
  a. arrhythmia.
  b. angina pectoris.
  c. atherosclerosis
  d. myocardial infarction.

_____ 5. Atherosclerosis is
  a. a narrowing of the arteries.
  b. the loss of elasticity of the arteries.
  c. another name for heart attack.
  d. characterized by a crushing pain in the chest.

_____ 6. Arteriosclerosis is
  a. a narrowing of the arteries.
  b. the loss of elasticity of the arteries.
  c. another name for heart attack.
  d. characterized by a crushing pain in the chest.

_____ 7. After feeling a crushing pain in the chest and difficulty in breathing, Roscoe went to a cardiologist who found no damage to Roscoe's myocardium. Roscoe was probably diagnosed as having
  a. a heart attack.
  b. a myocardial infarction.
  c. a stroke.
  d. angina pectoris.

159

_____ 8. Restriction of blood flow to the brain results in
    a. a stroke.
    b. an embolism.
    c. angina pectoris.
    d. a myocardial infarction.

_____ 9. Which of these blood pressure readings would be normal for an adult?
    a. systolic pressure of 120; diastolic pressure of 70
    b. diastolic pressure of 120; systolic pressure of 70
    c. diastolic pressure of 150; systolic pressure of 110
    d. systolic pressure of 150; diastolic pressure of 110

_____ 10. Which of these would be the best predictor of cardiovascular disease?
    a. Type A behavior pattern
    b. high levels of high-density lipoprotein
    c. being 15 pounds overweight
    d. high blood pressure

_____ 11. During the past 40 years, the death rate from cardiovascular disease in the United States has
    a. dropped dramatically.
    b. remained about the same.
    c. increased slightly.
    d. increased sharply.

_____ 12. The decline in the rate of first heart attacks strongly suggests that the overall drop in cardiovascular mortality
    a. is a temporary phenomenon.
    b. is due to improved medical procedures.
    c. results at least partially from changes in lifestyle.
    d. results from lower rates of compliance.

_____ 13. Which of these nations has recently experienced the highest rate of deaths from heart disease?
    a. Russia
    b. The United States
    c. Finland
    d. New Zealand

_____ 14. A risk factor for heart disease is
    a. any known cause of heart disease.
    b. any condition that predicts heart disease.
    c. any condition that results from heart disease.
    d. any condition that results in a decline in rate of heart disease.

_____ 15. Which of these factors is most clearly an inherent risk factor for cardiovascular disease?
   a. gender
   b. a high fat diet
   c. hostility
   d. hypertension

_____ 16. Which of these ethnic groups has the highest rates of cardiovascular mortality?
   a. Asian Americans
   b. European Americans
   c. Hispanic Americans
   d. African Americans

_____ 17. The strongest inherent risk factor for cardiovascular disease (and many others) is
   a. family history.
   b. smoking.
   c. advancing age.
   d. gender.

_____ 18. The strongest physiological risk factor for cardiovascular death is
   a. gender.
   b. smoking.
   c. Type A behavior pattern.
   d. hypertension.

_____ 19. HDL can be raised through
   a. exercise.
   d. decreased consumption of alcohol.
   c. quitting smoking.
   d. a diet high in saturated fats.

_____ 20. Total cholesterol
   a. is a better predictor of heart disease than the ratio of total cholesterol to HDL.
   b. is not reliably related to heart disease for older people.
   c. does not seem to be a risk factor for heart disease among children.
   d. both a and b are true.

_____ 21. Which of these people's cholesterol ratings places him at the highest risk for heart disease?
   a. Jerry, with a total cholesterol to HDL ratio is 7.0 to 1.0
   b. Bill, with a total cholesterol to HDL ratio is 3.5 to 1.
   c. Warren, with a total cholesterol to HDL ratio is 1.0 to 1.0.
   d. Kevin, with a total cholesterol to HDL ratio is 3.0 to 1.0.

_____ 22. Smoking, a known risk factor for lung cancer,
   a. is not a risk factor for heart disease.
   b. is a risk factor for heart disease for men but not for women.
   c. is a risk factor for heart disease for women but not for men.
   d. is a strong risk for heart disease for both men and women.

_____ 23. Celina, a manager of a retail clothing store, wants to reduce her risk for cardiovascular disease. She is 28 years old, about 15 pounds over her ideal weight, smokes a pack of cigarettes a day, drinks moderately, and has no family history of heart disease. Celina's best course of action would be to
   a. lose 20 pounds.
   b. stop smoking.
   c. stop drinking alcohol.
   d. quit her job.
   e. stop eating foods cooked in polyunsaturated fats.

_____ 24. Celina decides that she will start to take a low-dose aspirin every day to lower her risk for CVD. Her decision is based on the evidence that aspirin
   a. will lower her cholesterol.
   b. will lower her blood pressure.
   c. will reduce inflammation.
   d. will reduce her carbohydrate cravings and help her lower her weight.

_____ 25. Although obesity may not be an independent risk factor for cardiovascular disease, it is often related to
   a. hypertension.
   b. a sedentary life style.
   c. high cholesterol levels.
   d. all of the above.

_____ 26. High levels of depression
   a. seem to protect both men and women from heart disease.
   b. relate to the development of heart disease but not to its progression.
   c. relate to the progression of heart disease but not to its development.
   d. relate to both the development and progression of heart disease.

_____ 27. What component of the original Type A behavior pattern has received more support than the overall Type A concept?
   a. state anxiety
   b. a sense of time urgency
   c. hostility
   d. a strong sense of competition

_____ 28. The toxic component of hostility may be
    a. repressed hostility.
    b. repressed anxiety.
    c. expressed anger.
    d. interpersonal trust.

_____ 29. For most men, being _____ and having _____ is a strong risk for heart disease.
    a. married . . . a white-collar job
    b. unemployed . . . more than three children
    c. a college graduate . . . a high income
    d. single . . . little social support

_____ 30. Preventing heart disease is preferable to curing the disease. Which of these factors could be an effective way of preventing heart disease?
    a. stopping smoking
    c. limiting one's dietary fat to no more than 60% of one's caloric intake
    c. avoiding situations that may create anxiety
    d. lowering LDL levels

_____ 31. Dean Ornish and his colleges suggest that a diet with 30% of calories from fat
    a. may protect against the development of coronary artery damage.
    b. can reverse coronary artery damage without surgery.
    c. both a and b.
    d. neither a nor b.

_____ 32. Avery has experienced a heart attack, which left both he and his wife Lacey fearful about resuming sexual relations. They should know that such fears
    a. are uncommon among heart patients.
    b. are more common among female heart attack patients.
    c. are not justified by research.
    d. are justified, because many heart patients die during sexual relations.

Key Terms

Define each of the following:

arteriosclerosis —

atherosclerosis —

cardiovascular disease —

essential hypertension —

high-density lipoprotein —

low-density lipoprotein —

myocardial infarction —

stroke —

triglycerides —

Matching

Match the following:

1. arteries

   a. leading physiological risk factor for heart attack

2. HDL

   b. chronic inflammation that raises the risk for CVD

3. metabolic syndrome

   c. carry oxygenated blood to the heart muscle.

4. coronary arteries

   d. problems in glucose metabolism, excess abdominal fat, and high blood pressure

5. periodontal disease

   e. inherent risk factor for CVD

6. hypertension

   f. carry oxygenated blood to the body

7. myocardial infarction

   g. "good" cholesterol

8. Finland

   h. has an increasing rate of CVD

9. advancing age and family history

   i. has a declining rate of CVD

10. Russia

   j. heart attack

1. _____ 2. _____ 3. _____ 4. _____ 5. _____

6. _____ 7. _____ 8. _____ 9. _____ 10. _____

Evolution of the Type A Concept

Research on the toxic components of the Type A behavior pattern has evolved from the global pattern to more specific elements. Fill in the missing components in the following figure, arranging your answers so that the last item is the one that prompted further research.

Type A behavior pattern =

Concerned with _____ and the acquisition of _____ , exaggerated sense of _____ , competitiveness, and

_____

Suspiciousness, _____ _____ mistrust of others, and _____

Experience of _____ . _____ of anger

Essay Questions

1. Trace the development of the Type A behavior pattern to its current status.

2. Clint is a 35-year-old man who wants to lower his risk of developing cardiovascular disease. Give him some advice.

Let's Get Personal—
Will Cardiovascular Disease Happen to You?

Do you believe that you will develop cardiovascular disease? Recall that more than 30% of deaths in the United States are due to cardiovascular disease, so you are probably more likely to develop cardiovascular disease (CVD) than any other life-threatening disease. If you are a college student in your 20s, this possibility may seem very remote because cardiovascular disease is associated with middle-aged and elderly adults. The processes that result in CVD, however, begin during youth, and you may be building your risks right now.

What risk factors for CVD do you have? Answering the following questions will help you understand how this family of diseases can affect you.

Do you know your blood pressure, and is it in the normal range?

Do you eat a high-fat diet—one that is more than 30% of calories come from fat?

Do you eat five or more servings of fruits and vegetables per day?

What is your total cholesterol level?

Is your ratio of total cholesterol to high-density lipoprotein in the desirable range?

Do you smoke?

Do you follow a regular exercise program that gives you aerobic benefits?

Do many things anger you, and do you interpret the action of others as intentionally annoying?

Do you express your anger in ways that increase cardiovascular risks, such a yelling?

When you are angry, do you try to suppress your anger rather than expressing it?

Do you use stimulant drugs such as amphetamines or cocaine?

Although few young people die of cardiovascular disease, many have habits that will lead to CVD. If you believe that heart disease will not happen to you, the odds may not be in your favor.

Answers

Fill in the Rest of the Story

I.   blood; arteries; veins

I.A.   heart; coronary; atherosclerosis; arteriosclerosis

I.B.   plaque; coronary heart disease; ischemic; angina pectoris; heart attack

I.C.   brain; blood (oxygen)

I.D.   systolic; diastolic; hypertension; essential

II.   declined (decreased)

II.A.   lifestyle; first; smoking

II.B.   Soviet Union

III.   Framingham; causation

III.A. genetic; 10; 60; small; ethnic; twofold (double)

III.B. hypertension; cholesterol; High; low; high-density lipoprotein; saturated; diabetes; inflammation

III.C. smoking; positively; antioxidants; fruits; vegetables; activity; childhood

III.D. income; all-cause; social support; quality (satisfaction); depression; progression; cynical; anger; expression, reactivity; African; suppress

IV.   behaviors

IV.A. optimistic bias; unaware; sodium (salt): diet; expressing

IV.B. rehabilitation; Depressed; exercise; lifestyle; weight

Multiple Choice

1.	d	9.	a	17.	c	25.	d
2.	d	10.	d	18.	d	26.	d
3.	b	11.	a	19.	a	27.	c
4.	d	12.	c	20.	b	28.	c
5.	a	13.	a	21.	a	29.	d
6.	b	14.	b	22.	d	30.	a
7.	d	15.	a	23.	b	31.	a
8.	a	16.	d	24.	c	32.	c

Matching

1.	f	2.	g	3.	d	4.	c	5.	b
6.	a	7.	j	8.	i	9.	e	10.	h

Good points to include in your essay answers:

1. A. The concept of the Type A behavior pattern
    1. Originated by cardiologists Friedman and Rosenman.
    2. Included a pattern of behavior characteristic of coronary patients, including time pressure, competition, concern with money, impatience, and hostility.
    B. Initial support for the Type A concept was not confirmed, and the notion that global Type A behavior pattern as a risk for CVD faded.
    C. Hostility is a component of the Type A behavior pattern, and research focused on cynical hostility as a risk factor for CVD.
    D. Anger became a topic of research interest concerning cardiovascular risk.
    1. Both suppressed and expressed anger may increase the risk, but expressed anger is the greater risk.
    2. The CVD risk for anger may apply only to some people and not all people.

2. A. Clint's risks depend on his inherent risk factors as well as his behaviors and habits, but he can lower his risks by changing his behavior.
    B. Clint should know his blood pressure and try to either keep his blood pressure in the normal range or bring his hypertension back toward normal.
    1. If he is overweight, losing weight can lower his blood pressure.
    2. Complying to blood pressure medication can be important.
    C. Clint should not smoke.
    D. Clint should eat a diet low in fat and high in fiber in an attempt to maintain or attain serum cholesterol level below 200.
    1. If his cholesterol level is high, he may not be able to lower it through diet alone.
    2. He should be concerned about the ratio of total cholesterol to high-density lipoprotein (HDL), striving for a high HDL count.
    E. Clint should consider taking an anti-inflammatory drug regularly.
    F. Clint should try to maintain an overall positive mood and avoid or manage tendencies toward depression.
    G. Clint should express any anger in with a slow, soft voice and try to avoid any expression of cynical hostility.

CHAPTER 10
Behavioral Factors in Cancer

Learning Objectives

After studying Chapter 10, you should be able to

1. Define cancer.

2. Discuss the types of cancer with increasing and decreasing rates.

3. Distinguish between risk factors beyond personal control and those that arise from behavior and lifestyle.

4. Evaluate the relative importance of the behavioral and psychosocial risk factors for cancer.

5. Explain the challenges of living with cancer.

Fill in the Rest of the Story

I. What Is Cancer?

Cancer is a group of diseases characterized by the presence of _____ cells that grow and spread beyond control. Neoplastic cells can be either _____ or malignant. Malignant tumors _____, that is, they invade and destroy surrounding tissue. Malignant growths can be divided into four main groups—carcinomas, or cancerous cells of the _____, stomach lining, and mucous membrane; _____, or cancerous cells of the connective tissue such as bone, muscles, and cartilage; _____ or cancers that originate in the blood or blood-forming cells, such as bone marrow; and lymphomas, or cancer of the _____ system.

II. The Changing Rates of Cancer Deaths

During the past 15 years, cancer death rates in the United States have _____, a situation due in part to changes in diet and a decline in _____ rates and in part to earlier diagnosis and improved treatments.

A. Cancers with Decreasing Death Rates

Cancer of the lungs, breast, _____, and colon/rectum account for about half of all cancer deaths in the United States. _____ cancer accounts for about 28% of all cancer deaths and about 15% of all cancer cases per year—figures that reveal the _____ of lung cancer. Lung cancer deaths among men are currently _____, whereas those of women are beginning to level off. Breast cancer has a high _____ but not as high a death rate for women in the United States. Prostate cancer has a high incidence among men in the United States but not the highest _____ rate. The second leading cause of cancer deaths in the United States is _____ cancer. Incidence and morality rates for this cancer vary widely by ethnic background, with _____ Americans much more likely to be diagnosed with colorectal cancer than other ethnic groups. Death rates from _____ cancer have dropped from being the leading cause of cancer deaths for both women and men to having a very low mortality rate.

B. Cancers with Increasing Incidence and Mortality Rates

Liver cancer is quite lethal, with a death rate nearly _____ as high as its incidence rate. Melanoma is a potentially fatal form of _____ cancer that is increasing among men but not among women.

III. Cancer Risks Beyond Personal Control

Inherent and environmental conditions are mostly beyond personal control and may contribute to the development of cancer.

A. Inherent Risk Factors for Cancer

African Americans have an increased risk of death from cancer, which may be attributable to _____ status rather than ethnicity. As with heart disease, the greatest risk factor for cancer is advancing _____; the older people become, the greater their chances of dying of cancer. Genetic factors play a role in _____ cancer in women who inherit a mutation in the _____ gene. A more common genetic influence is an interaction between environmental or behavioral risks and genes, which is called a genetic _____.

B. Environmental Risk Factors for Cancer

Environmental factors include exposure to radiation, _____ pesticides, and other chemicals. These environmental risks are quite small and difficult to estimate. Working in a _____ power plant has a slightly greater association with cancer, but living near such a plant does not.

IV. Behavioral Risks for Cancer

Although heredity plays a role in the development of cancer, about two thirds of all cancer deaths in the United States are associated with smoking and _____.

A. Smoking

Male cigarette smokers have about a 23 times greater risk of death from _____ _____ than do nonsmokers. In addition, the more cigarettes a person smokes, the greater the chances of developing cancer; that is, the risk is a _____-_____ risk. Many smokers believe that the negative effects of smoking affect other smokers but not themselves; that is, they possess an _____ _____ that tends to perpetuate their risky behavior. When smoking is combined with exposure to air pollution and building materials such as asbestos, the risk of lung cancer becomes more than additive—it becomes _____.

B. Diet

Diet may account for as much 33% of cancer deaths. Eating spoiled foods or foods _____ with toxins increases the risk. Some foods may offer protection, but identifying specific foods or nutrients has proven difficult. A healthy diet, especially one high in fruits and _____, decreases the risk of several types of cancer. In general, eating a healthy diet is more beneficial than taking _____ to receive nutrients.

C. Alcohol

Alcohol is probably a _____ risk factor for cancer, but it may have a synergistic effect when combined with _____, placing some heavy drinkers at a much greater risk for cancer of the larynx.

D. Sedentary Lifestyle

Physical activity may offer some protection against cancer. Moderate exercise is related to lower rates of _____ cancer in men and women and _____ cancer in women.

E. Ultraviolet Light

The most common form of cancer in the United States is _____ cancer, but death rates from this cancer are relatively low. However, one form of skin cancer—malignant _____ has a high death rate. Exposure to ultraviolet light also has benefits because it prompts the body to produce _____ _____.

F. Sexual Behavior

Sexual behavior plays a role in cancers that result from AIDS, such as _____ sarcoma and non-Hodgkin's _____. For women, early age at first _____ and a large number of _____ _____ increase the risks for cancer of the cervix, vagina, and ovaries. Conversely, early _____ and childbirth may offer some protection against breast cancer.

G. Psychosocial Risk Factors in Cancer

Evidence for a relationship between psychosocial risk factors and cancer is not strong. Negative _____ and repression of emotion show some relationship.

V. Living with Cancer

More than a million Americans are diagnosed with cancer each year.

A. Problems with Medical Treatments for Cancer

Cancer patients who undergo _____ are likely to experience distress, rejection, and fears, and they often receive less emotional support than other surgery patients. Many patients who receive _____ therapy anticipate their treatment with fear and anxiety, fearing hair loss, burns, nausea, vomiting, fatigue, and sterility. Chemotherapy is also frequently accompanied by many of these same unpleasant side effects.

B. Adjusting to a Diagnosis of Cancer

Most cancer patients find difficulty in adjusting to their diagnosis. They are likely to experience feelings of fear, anxiety, and _____ as a result of their diagnosis and treatment for cancer. Separating depression and cancer is difficult, and those with severe depression may experience more rapid _____ of their cancer.

C. Social Support for Cancer Patents

The support of spouses, family members, and friends can help cancer patients by increasing their access to _____ support, strengthening a sense of personal control, fostering self-esteem, and boosting their feelings of optimism. The importance of social support has led to the creation of _____ _____, but not all cancer patient benefit from such groups.

D. Psychotherapy with Cancer Patients

Psychotherapy with cancer patients is oriented toward improving their quality of life, reducing _____, and helping them develop healthy behaviors. Although psychotherapy can help cancer patients improve their _____ of life, research has failed to show its power to increase _____ time.

177

Multiple Choice Questions

_____ 1. Unlike benign tumors, malignant tumors
   a. attack only tissue cells.
   b. can metastasize.
   c. grow more slowly.
   d. cannot metastasize.

_____ 2. Cancerous cells of the skin, stomach lining, and mucous membranes are called
   a. sarcomas.
   b. carcinomas.
   c. leukemia.
   d. lymphomas.

_____ 3. During the past 15 years, cancer death rates in the United States have increased for which of these sites?
   a. breast
   b. prostate
   c. lung
   d. colon/rectum
   e. none of the above

_____ 4. Lung cancer accounts for about 28% of cancer deaths and about 15% of all cancer diagnoses per year. These numbers suggest that
   a. lung cancer death rates are increasing.
   b. lung cancer death rates are decreasing.
   c. lung cancer prevalence is higher than its incidence.
   d. lung cancer is a deadly disease.

_____ 5. Among women, other than skin cancer, _____ cancer has the highest incidence but not the highest death rate of cancers in the United States.
   a. breast
   b. lung
   c. stomach
   d. colorectal

_____ 6. The second leading cause of cancer *deaths* in the United States is _____ cancer.
   a. stomach
   b. prostate
   c. breast
   d. lung
   e. colorectal

_____ 7. Inherent risk factors for cancer include
   a. advancing age.
   b. drinking alcohol.
   c. a diet high in fiber.
   d. smoking.

_____ 8. Which ethnic group has the highest rate of cancer deaths?
   a. European American
   b. Asian American
   c. Hispanic American
   d. African American

_____ 9. In general, inherent and environmental risk factors for cancer
   a. are much weaker than behavioral risk factors.
   b. account for about 50% of all cancers deaths.
   c. are much more difficult to treat than lung cancer.
   d. All of the above are true.
   e. None of the above is true.

_____ 10. Which of these factors is the strongest environmental risk factor for cancer?
   a. alcohol consumption
   b. living near a nuclear power plant
   c. working in a nuclear power plant
   d. working in a fast food store

_____ 11. Cancer death rates are highest for
   a. children below age 12.
   b. adolescents and young adults.
   c. middle-aged adults.
   d. older people.

_____ 12. Which of these factors has contributed most to cancer death rates in the United States during the past 50 years?
   a. pesticides
   b. carcinogens in the drinking water
   c. sexual practices
   d. cigarette smoking

_____ 13. Of the factors listed, which represents the highest risk for cancer in the United States?
   a. alcohol
   b. diet
   c. ultraviolet light
   d. sexual practices

179

_____ 14. Michelle, a 20-year-old college student, wants to do whatever is possible to avoid cancer. What research results are important for her to understand?
  a. evidence that "natural" foods with no preservatives decrease cancer risk
  b. evidence that salt-cured foods decrease cancer risk
  c. evidence that a high protein diet, featuring meat and dairy products, offers protection against cancer
  d. evidence that a healthy diet with lots of fruits and vegetables offers more protection than taking supplements

_____ 15. During the past 75 years, stomach cancer death rates have dropped sharply. The primary reason for this decline is
  a. earlier detection of cancer growths.
  b. higher consumption of fruits and vegetables.
  c. use of refrigeration.
  d. the widespread use of dietary supplements.

_____ 16. Which cancer kills more women in the United States than any other type of cancer?
  a. lung cancer
  b. breast cancer
  c. stomach cancer
  d. cancer of the uterus

_____ 17. Which cancer kills more men in the United States than any other type of cancer?
  a. lung cancer
  b. prostrate cancer
  c. stomach cancer
  d. colon cancer

_____ 18. The most common type of cancer in the United States has a very low death rate; it is
  a. colon cancer.
  b. skin cancer.
  c. liver cancer.
  d. leukemia.

_____ 19. The ingredient in pizza that may offer some protection against cancer is (are)
  a. the tomato sauce.
  b. the mushrooms.
  c. the anchovies.
  d. the cheese.

_____20. Jace is considering a program of high-dose vitamins to protect against cancer. What is good advice to him?
   a. Make sure the vitamins are natural; synthesized nutrients are not protective.
   b. Taking only a multivitamin will offer protection; you don't need high levels of nutrients to obtain protection.
   c. Don't bother; the typical U.S. diet contains nutrients that offer protection.
   d. Consider changing your diet instead; obtaining nutrients through diet is a better strategy.

_____21. Alcohol
   a. is not a risk factor for cancer.
   b. is a strong risk factor for cancer.
   c. is generally a strong risk factor for cancer, but it effects are limited to colon cancer.
   d. is generally a weak risk factor for cancer, but it can have a synergistic effect with smoking that increases people's risk of laryngeal cancer.

_____22. Research on the relationship between a sedentary life style and various cancer sites has generally found that physical activity reduces several types of cancer. An exception to these findings is evidence that
   a. men who had worked many years on strenuous jobs have an increase in prostate cancer.
   b. men, but not women, who have engaged many years in leisure-time activities have low rates of colorectal cancer.
   c. women, but not men, who have engaged many years in leisure-time activities had low rates of colorectal cancer.
   d. physical activity seems to promote lung cancer in non-smokers.

_____23. In general, skin cancer risk in the United States is greatest for
   a. African Americans.
   b. Hispanic Americans.
   c. fair-skinned European Americans living in northern cities and towns.
   d. fair-skinned European Americans living in southern cities and towns.

_____24. Which of these factors is positively related to cancer of the cervix?
   a. late age at first intercourse
   b. high socioeconomic status
   c. having many sex partners
   d. having a first child late in life

_____25. Psychosocial risk factors for cancer
   a. are not as strong as behavioral factors.
   b. are stronger than inherent factors such as advancing age.
   c. are better predictors of cancer in women than in men.
   d. do not relate to the development of any type of cancer.

_____ 26. A diagnosis of cancer is most likely to result in
    a. suicide in about 30% of cases.
    b. expressions of anxiety and anger.
    c. severe and extended feelings of depression.
    d. a combination of each of these.

_____ 27. The type of social support that is most effective for cancer patients is
    a. support from spouses rather than from family.
    b. support from a support group.
    c. support that is helpful but yet not obvious.
    d. support that targets practical and not emotional distress.

_____ 28. One important difference between medical procedures for cancer and those for heart disease is that cancer treatments
    a. are much more expensive.
    b. result in fewer distressing side effects.
    c. result in more distressing side effects.
    d. are more likely to produce feelings of paranoia.

Key Terms

Define each of the following:

benign —

carcinogen —

carcinoma —

flavonols —

leukemia —

lymphoma —

metastasize —

neoplastic —

oncologist —

sarcoma —

Matching

Match the following:

1. metastasize	a.	cancer with the highest death rate
2. smoking	b.	interaction of alcohol and smoking
3. synergistic effect	c.	cancer of the connective tissue
4. negative emotionality	d.	invade and destroy surrounding tissue
5. lung cancer	e.	a leading behavioral risk for cancer
6. breast and prostate cancer	f.	nutrients that may protect against cancer
7. BRCA	g.	leading inherent risk factor for cancer
8. advancing age	h.	cancer with high incidence but lower mortality rate
9. flavonols	i.	genetic risk for cancer
10. sarcoma	j.	psychosocial risk factor for cancer

1. _____ 2. _____ 3. _____ 4. _____ 5. _____

6. _____ 7. _____ 8. _____ 9. _____ 10. _____

Changes in Cancer Rates

The following figures represent changes in several of the leading causes of cancer deaths over the past 70 years. Label the types of cancer deaths for men and for women.

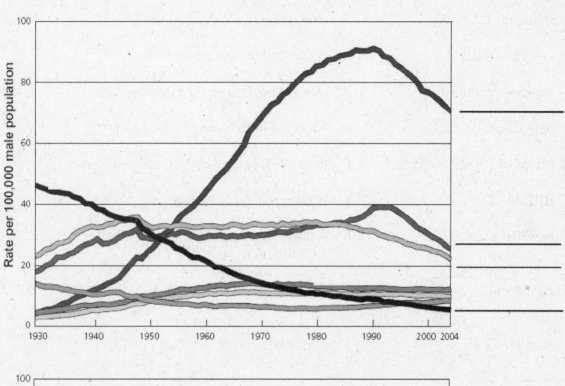

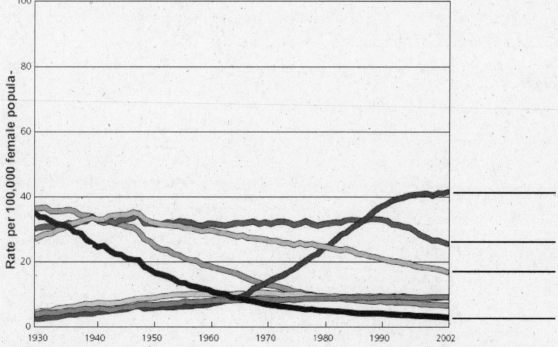

Essay Questions

1. Garland is a smoker who believes that air pollution is the major cause of lung cancer. Is his belief accurate, and what is probably responsible for his attitude?

2. Brittany wants to protect herself against cancer. What should she do?

Let's Get Personal—
Are You Increasing Your Risk?

Cancer is complex group of diseases, consisting of several different types of malignancies that affect a variety of body sites. The major risk factors for cancer are behaviors, and you may have habits that increase your risk. In addition, you may be at risk for cancer as a result of hereditary or environmental factors beyond your control. Although the research indicates that personal behaviors provide the biggest risks, people have trouble accepting that they are behaving in ways that are harmful.

To understand how your behavior may be raising your risk for cancer, choose a type of cancer for which your risk is elevated. If you do not know of any type for which you have an elevated risk, you may determine your risk by completing one of the brief cancer screenings offered by the American Cancer Society. Once you have chosen a type of cancer, research the risk factors that increase the chances of developing it, beginning with the information in your textbook. When you have discovered the risks, divide them into behavioral versus hereditary and environmental. Which type of risk factors raises the relative risk more? If the type of cancer you have researched is like most types, the behavioral risks are bigger, and you may be doing things that raise your risk.

Type of cancer:

How high is your risk compared to other people your age?

What are the behaviors that elevate the risk for this type of cancer?

What are the environmental and hereditary factors that elevate the risk?

Which type of factor increases the risk more dramatically—behavioral or environmental/hereditary?

How can you lower your risk?

Answers

Fill in the Rest of the Story

I. neoplastic (new); benign; metastasize; skin; sarcomas; leukemias; lymphatic

II. declined; smoking (cigarettes)

II.A. prostate; Lung; deadliness; declining; incidence; mortality (death); colorectal (colon/rectal); African; stomach

II.B. twice; skin

III.A. socioeconomic; age; breast; BRCA; predisposition

III.B. asbestos; nuclear

IV. diet

IV.A. lung cancer; dose-response; optimistic bias; synergistic

IV.B. contaminated; vegetables; supplements

IV.C. weak; cigarette smoking

IV.D. colon; breast

IV.E. skin; melanoma; vitamin D

IV.F. Kaposi's; lymphoma; intercourse; sexual partners; pregnancy

IV.G. emotionality

V.A. surgery; radiation

V.B. depression; progression

V.C. social; support groups

V.D. stress; quality; survival

Multiple Choice Answers

1. b	8. d	15. c	22. a
2. b	9. a	16. a	23. d
3. e	10. c	17. a	24. c
4. d	11. d	18. b	25. a
5. a	12. d	19. a	26. b
6. e	13. b	20. d	27. c
7. a	14. d	21. d	28. c

Matching

1. d	2. e	3. b	4. j	5. a
6. h	7. i	8. g	9. f	10. c

Good points to include in your essay answers:

1. A. Garland's belief is inaccurate. The threat from air pollution is minor in comparison with that from smoking.
    1. Smoking increases the risk for lung cancer about 23 times compared to nonsmokers.
    2. This link is the strongest for any behavior-illness pairing.
   B. Like Garland, smokers tend to have a perceived risk that is not as strong as the actual risk.
    1. This perception is the result of optimistic bias that makes smokers believe that the negative consequences of smoking will happen to other smokers but not to them.
    2. People who engage in risky behaviors have trouble acknowledging that their behavior places them at risk.

2. A. Alice probably cannot completely protect herself against cancer.
    1. Some cancers have a hereditary component.
    2. Many environmental factors relate to the development of cancer and avoiding all would be impossible.
   B. Alice can lower her risk in several ways.
    1. She should not smoke or use any other form of tobacco.
    2. She should avoid a high-fat diet and concentrate on increasing her intake of fruits, vegetables, and grains.
    3. She should avoid excessive drinking, especially in combination with smoking.
    4. She should participate in physical exercise.
    5. She should avoid sun exposure and should not try to develop a tan.
    6. She should avoid risky sexual behaviors, but she faces a dilemma.
        a. Early intercourse raises the risk for reproductive cancers.
        b. Early pregnancy decreases the risk for breast cancer.
    7. She should try to develop healthy strategies for expressing emotion and avoid focusing on negative emotions and events.

CHAPTER 11
Living with Chronic Illness

Learning Objectives

After studying Chapter 11, you should be able to

1. Analyze the impact of chronic illness on patients and their families.

2. Compare the processes of living with a chronic disease and facing death.

3. Describe the symptoms and physiological basis for Alzheimer's disease.

4. Identify the role of health psychologists in researching and treating Alzheimer's disease.

5. Distinguish the risks and treatment for Type 1 and Type 2 diabetes.

6. Explain how psychological factors may contribute to the development and management of diabetes.

7. Evaluate the theories of asthma.

8. Discuss how health psychologists contribute to the management of asthma.

9. Trace the four HIV/AIDS epidemics in the United States.

10. Contrast HIV infection in the United States with the worldwide epidemic.

11. Explain psychologists' role in the AIDS epidemic.

Fill in the Rest of the Story

I. The Impact of Chronic Illness

The diagnosis of a _____ illness may present a crisis or a transition, but such a diagnosis requires adaptation. Adjustment to the illness may change the way patients see themselves, produce financial strain, and disrupt established patterns of personal and social behaviors.

A. Impact on the Patient

Chronically ill people must cope with their symptoms and with the stresses of receiving treatment. Dealing with the health care system is often a _____ factor for people with chronic illness, partly because health care providers typically concentrate on the physical aspects of the illness and fail to provide help in coping with the long-term disruption of the patient's life. Support _____ can be valuable for people with

chronic illness, providing information as well as emotional support.

B. Impact on the Family

Chronic illness requires _____ for families as well as for individuals. For

families with chronically ill children, parents must adapt to their child's illness and manage

other family responsibilities. Chronically ill adults often require special care, and family

members are often _____, and this change alters the relationship. Feelings of

loss and _____ are common for individuals with chronic illness and for their

family members.

II. Living with Alzheimer's Disease

Alzheimer's disease is a degenerative disease of the _____ and a major source

of impairment among older people. Increasing _____ is the leading risk factor.

Two forms of the disease exist, an early-onset type that occurs before age 60 and a late-onset

type that begins after age 60. The more common of the two is the late-onset type, which seems to

be related to apolipoprotein ε, a _____ involved in cholesterol metabolism.

Symptoms of Alzheimer's disease include language problems, memory loss, confusion,

wandering, agitation and irritability, sleep disorders, depression, suspiciousness, incontinence,

sexual disorders, and loss of ability to perform routine self-care.

A. Helping the Patient

Alzheimer's disease is presently incurable, and drugs have only a limited ability to

control this illness. Several psychological interventions are used to minimize

disorientation, including the presentation of _____ stimulation and

interventions to help them cope with depression.

B. Helping the Family

The symptoms of Alzheimer disease are very distressing to family members who are

subjected to emotional outbursts, suspiciousness, anger, and agitation. As the disease

progresses, constant care is required because the Alzheimer's patient may

_____ away from home at all times of the day or night. Psychosocial

interventions such as _____ groups often help caregivers cope with the

strain of living with an Alzheimer's patient.

III. Adjusting to Diabetes

With increased obesity among American youth, many children as young as 8 or 9 years old

are now developing _____ _____ diabetes. Both Type 1 and Type 2

diabetes require changes in lifestyle, including the frequent monitoring of

_____ _____ and strict compliance to treatment. Type 1 diabetes

requires insulin injections as well as adherence to a _____ regimen. Type 2

diabetes does not ordinarily require insulin injections, but it does demand strict compliance to a

rigid dietary regimen, regular medical visits, and routine _____.

A. The Physiology of Diabetes

Diabetes mellitus is a disorder caused by an _____ deficiency. The

islet cells of the pancreas produce _____, which stimulates the release

of glucose, and insulin, which allows cells to use glucose. If the islet cells do not produce

adequate insulin, excessive _____ accumulates in the blood and urine.

Patients' inability to regulate blood sugar often causes diabetics to develop other health

problems such as _____ disease, retina damage, and kidney diseases.

B. The Impact of Diabetes

The diagnosis of Type 1 diabetes affects both the child and the parents. The child is

labeled as sick or different, and faces a _____ of coping with a chronic

disease. Although Type 2 diabetes does not usually require insulin injections, it does demand

lifestyle changes such as diet and medication. Some people with diabetes refuse to

_____ to their treatment regimen, which creates risks for the

development of health problems.

C. Health Psychology's Involvement with Diabetes

Some psychology research has concentrated on ways that diabetics

_____ their disease and how these conceptualizations affect self-care,

the effects of stress on glucose metabolism, and reasons for noncompliance. Research

indicates that _____ affects both the development of diabetes and glucose

metabolism. However, a major problem is adhering to the required testing, diet, and exercise

regimen. Much of the _____ research has centered on children and

adolescents, who are particularly poor at complying with the medical and behavioral regimen

required for controlling their blood sugar.

IV. The Impact of Asthma

About 8.5% of adults in the United States have asthma, but the rate is the highest for

_____ Americans and for children and adolescents between ages 5 and

17. The death rate from asthma is not high, but it is the largest cause of disability among

_____.

A. The Disease of Asthma

Asthma is a chronic disease that causes constriction of the _____

tubes, preventing air from passing freely. People with asthma may go for long periods of

time without any problems in breathing, but the condition can return at any time. Asthma

may be due to a genetic vulnerability that makes the immune system of some infants respond

with an _____ reaction to certain substances in the environment. Another

view, the hygiene hypothesis, holds that asthma is a result of the

_____ that has become common in modern societies, with results for

the immune system and its response to bacteria and dirt.

B. Managing Asthma

Managing asthma requires a variety of medications as well as learning personal

_____ and avoiding them. Drugs for asthma often have unpleasant side

effects, such as _____ gain and lack of energy, conditions that make adherence difficult. Asthma attacks can cause respiratory failure, which may be fatal, so

people with asthma benefit by learning appropriate self care.

V. Dealing with HIV and AIDS

Acquired immune deficiency syndrome is a disorder produced by the

_____ _____ _____ (HIV), which

causes the immune system to lose its effectiveness and leaves the body defenseless against

bacterial, viral, fungal, parasitic, cancerous, and other _____

diseases.

A. Incidence and Mortality Rates for HIV/AIDS

Since 1993, death rates from AIDS in the United States have dramatically

_____ because people who are HIV positive are now

_____ _____ and people at high risk are making

changes in their lifestyle to lower risk.

B. The HIV and AIDS Epidemics

The four HIV/AIDS epidemics are (1) male-male sexual contact, (2)

_____ _____ use, (3) heterosexual contact, and (4)

transmission from _____ to _____. Of these four

epidemics, the one with the greatest decline in mortality in the United States is male-male

sexual contact. Worldwide, _____ contact is the leading cause of HIV

infection.

C. Symptoms of HIV and AIDS

HIV typically progresses over a decade or more from infection to AIDS. During the first

phase after infection, people often experience symptoms similar to _____.

The next phase shows no symptoms, but the infected person's _____ system

is being destroyed. When the infected person's CD4+ cell count falls to the point that

_____ infections begin, symptoms of swollen lymph nodes, fever, fatigue,

night sweats, loss of appetite, and loss of weight occur. Additional decreases in CD4+ cells

195

lead to a diagnosis of _____ and other infections, including *Pneumocystis carninii* pneumonia and Kaposi's sarcoma.

D. The Transmission of HIV

The main routes of HIV infection are from person to person through

_____ contact, from mother to child during pregnancy or birth, and from direct contact with blood or blood products. The largest number of HIV infections in the United States is still through _____ to _____ sexual contact, with anal intercourse being especially risky for the receptive partner. The sharing of unsterilized needles by _____ drug users allows the direct transmission of infected blood from one person to another and is the _____ most frequent source of HIV infection among men and women in the United States. The leading source of HIV infection in Africa, and the leading source of HIV infection among women in the United States, is _____ _____. Unsafe sexual behaviors are situational, and many people do not feel comfortable in asking a partner to use a

_____.

E. Psychologists' Role in the AIDS Epidemic

Psychologists have played several roles in controlling the AIDS epidemic, including investigating the behavioral aspects of AIDS, counseling with HIV patients, changing _____-_____ behaviors, and helping patients adopt healthier lifestyles. They help people change risky behaviors, such as sharing _____ with an infected person and having _____ sexual contact with an infected person.

VI. Facing Death

People prefer a long life, but they also express preferences to be in control over the end of their lives and to die a "_____ _____."

A. Adjusting to Terminal Illness

Elizabeth Kübler-Ross proposed that adjusting to terminal illness occurred through five stages. Research has confirmed that people experience the reactions she proposed but not the _____ of the stages. A more useful conceptualization is the _____ role, which is an extension of the sick role. The key elements for the dying role are settling practical, _____, and personal issues. A lack of access to palliative care represents a barrier to fulfilling the dying role.

B. Grieving

People who are dying often experience feelings similar to those of their loved ones— _____ and _____. A process of adaptation occurs during _____, but that process does not take the form of a fixed sequence of stages. Rather, people experience _____ emotions, and adapting takes time.

Multiple Choice Questions

_____ 1. Ronald Reagan, the story at the beginning of this chapter, had many symptoms of Alzheimer's disease, including
   a. elevated blood pressure.
   b. memory loss.
   c   compulsive neatness.
   d. miserliness.

_____ 2. The diagnosis of chronic illness may be interpreted as a crisis or as a psychosocial transition, but both models stress the importance of
   a. negative coping.
   b. optimism.
   c. adaptation.
   d. experience.

_____ 3. Chronic illnesses persist over a period of time. Most people with a chronic illness
   a. understand this fact.
   b. attempt to make their lives as normal as possible.
   c. will eventually be cured of their illness.
   d. both b and c.

_____ 4. The chronic illness that is usually the most disruptive to families is
   a. heart disease.
   b. cancer.
   c. AIDS.
   d. Alzheimer's disease.

_____ 5. For chronically ill people, the difficulties in interacting with the health care system come from
   a. their own attitudes of hopelessness and helplessness.
   b. the pessimistic attitudes that health care providers have toward the chronically ill.
   c. the supportive attitudes of families.
   d. both a and b.

_____ 6. Eileen has received a diagnosis of breast cancer. She believes that her treatment will not be a problem, and she is certain that her treatment will be successful in eradicating her cancer. These very optimistic expectancies
   a. will interfere with her treatment.
   b. will pose problems when she enters the health care system.
   c. may be positive factors in adapting to her illness.
   d. both a and b.

_____ 7. The risk for which of the following diseases increases sharply with age?
   a. Type I diabetes
   b. acquired immune deficiency syndrome
   c. leukemia
   d. Alzheimer's disease

_____ 8. Which of these is most likely to be a symptom of Alzheimer's disease?
   a. high blood pressure
   b. wandering and sleep disorders
   c. high cholesterol
   d. increased memory for recent events

_____ 9. Vernon, a 72-year-old man, has been wandering about his neighborhood at unusual hours of the day. He seems both confused and agitated. For no apparent reason, he strikes out at his wife verbally, though he has never hit her. He has some awareness that his memory is not as good as it once was, and this knowledge frustrates him. These symptoms best describe
   a. AIDS.
   b. Alzheimer's disease.
   c. attention deficit disorder.
   d. Kaposi's sarcoma.

_____ 10. Which of these factors may offer some amount of protection against advancing Alzheimer's disease?
    a. having an occupation that keeps a person cognitively active
    b. not drinking any alcohol
    c. drinking water with high levels of aluminum
    d. having Type 2 diabetes

_____ 11. Diabetes is a disorder caused by a(n) _____ deficiency.
    a. white blood cell
    b. insulin
    c. red blood cell
    d. sodium

_____ 12. Which type of diabetes does NOT usually require insulin injections?
    a. Type 1
    b. Type 2
    c. neither Type 1 nor Type 2
    d. both Type 1 and Type 2

_____ 13. Most adults who develop diabetes
    a. are men.
    b. are thin.
    c. require insulin injections.
    d. none of the above.

_____ 14. Until a few years ago, Type 2 diabetes was called adult-onset diabetes. What prompted the change in terminology to Type 2?
    a. Fewer people have been diagnosed with Type 1 diabetes.
    b. Fewer people have been diagnosed with Type 2 diabetes.
    c. Type 2 diabetes has become increasingly common among chidden.
    d. Type 1 diabetes has become increasingly common among adults.

_____ 15. A serious problem for diabetic adolescents is
    a. lack of time to do school work.
    b. obesity.
    c. adherence to the required regimen.
    d. increased risk for colon cancer.

_____ 16. Asthma is a chronic condition found most frequently in
    a. infants.
    b. children ages 5 to 17.
    c. middle-aged men.
    d. women ages 70 to 85.

_____17. The hygiene hypothesis suggests that asthma may result from
   a. low blood sugar.
   b. high blood pressure.
   c. an unsterile environment.
   d. a clean environment.

_____18. The United States has four HIV/AIDS epidemics. Which one is NOT one of the four?
   a. injection drug use
   b. male-male sexual contact
   c. blood transfusions
   d. male-female sexual contact

_____19. Since the mid-1990s, the death rate from AIDS has
   a. increased sharply.
   b. increased gradually.
   c. remained about the same.
   d. decreased sharply.

_____20. Currently, more than _____ people worldwide are infected with the HIV virus.
   a. one million
   b. five million
   c. 17 million
   d. 40 million

_____21. During the past decade, the incidence of AIDS has dropped, but mortality has dropped even more. This suggests that
   a. the prevalence of AIDS has also greatly decreased.
   b. the prevalence of AIDS is unaffected by these two findings.
   c. people are living longer after being diagnosed with AIDS.
   d. people are dying sooner after being diagnosed with AIDS.

_____22. During the past decade, the largest decline in the proportion of HIV cases was among
   a. gay men.
   b. African American women.
   c. injection drug users.
   d. European American women

_____23. The recent decline in AIDS mortality in the United States is due to a
   a. shorter survival time for AIDS patients.
   b. decline in the incidence of AIDS.
   c. decline in the incidence rates of HIV infection among heterosexual women.
   d. an increase in the incidence of HIV infection among heterosexual men.

_____24. A description of the typical person who is HIV positive in the United States includes
    a. being male.
    b. being female.
    c. being Asian American.
    d. high socioeconomic status.

_____25. HIV infection progresses over a decade. The first symptoms include
    a. CD4+ T-lymphocyte cell falls to a count of less than 200.
    b. a period of latency in which the person experiences few, if any symptoms.
    c. symptoms of fever, sore throat, skin rash, and headache.
    d. a cluster of symptoms, including swollen lymph nodes, fever, fatigue, night sweats, and loss of appetite.

_____26. The LEAST likely mode of HIV transmission would be
    a. receiving a blood transfusion from someone infected with HIV.
    b. having sexual intercourse with someone who is infected.
    c. sharing eating utensils with someone who is infected.
    d. sharing injection needles with someone who is infected.

_____27. All of the following are associated with unprotected sexual contact among gay men except
    a. heavy use of alcohol.
    b. heavy drug use.
    c. being 35 years old or older.
    d. willingness to engage in other risky behaviors.

_____28. During the decade from 1995 to 2005, the incidence of HIV infection in the United States increased fastest for
    a. female injection drug users.
    b. male injection drug users.
    c. male-female sexual contact.
    d. male-male sexual contact.

_____29. Elizabeth Kübler-Ross proposed that individuals diagnosed with a terminal illness go through stages in dying. Research
    a. fails to confirm that a sequences of stages occurs.
    b. has confirmed the sequence of stages she proposed.
    c. indicates that most people who are terminally ill do not ever reach acceptance.
    d. indicates large differences in the stages, depending on the age of the dying person.

_____30. Which of the following represents an alternative conceptualization of the process of dying from the one proposed by Elizabeth Kübler-Ross?
    a. the diathesis-stress model
    b. the dying role
    c. the stages of change model
    d. the concept of social support

Key Terms

Define each of the following:

Alzheimer's disease —

asthma —

HIV —

hygiene hypothesis —

insulin —

pancreas —

Type 1 diabetes —

Type 2 diabetes —

Matching

Match the following:

1. *pneumocystis carninii* pneumonia

2. Type 1 diabetes

3. apolipoprotein ɛ4

4. Type 2 diabetes

5. asthma

6. anger, denial, bargaining

7. cardiovascular disease, kidney disease, and retinal damage

8. hygiene hypothesis

9. islet cells of the pancreas

10. heterosexual sex

a. reactions to terminal illness

b. insulin production

c. insulin-dependent

d. risks associated with diabetes

e. AIDS

f. largest cause of disability among children

g. risk for Alzheimer's disease

h. leading mode of HIV infection worldwide

i. noninsulin-dependent

j. asthma

1. _____ 2. _____ 3. _____ 4. _____ 5. _____

6. _____ 7. _____ 8. _____ 9. _____ 10. _____

Gender, Ethnicity, and HIV Infection

To better understand the impact of HIV infection on women and men in various ethnic groups, fill in the missing information in this figure.

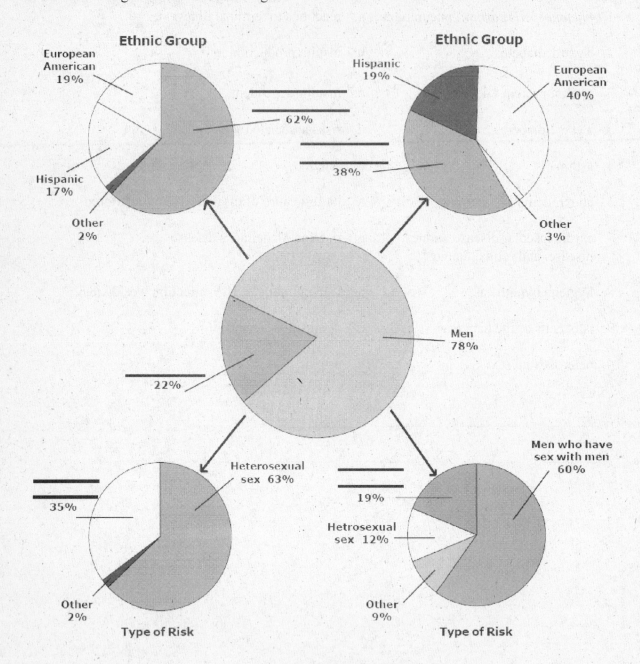

Essay Questions

1. What psychological factors are important in the management of diabetes?

2. Evaluate the statement: "With the new drugs developed to treat AIDS, psychologists will play a less important role in the AIDS epidemic."

Let's Get Personal—
How Chronic Illness Changed My Family

To better understand the impact of chronic illness on families, interview someone who has a chronic condition or someone who has lived with a person with a chronic illness. Chronic illness is very common, so finding someone who has lived with chronic illness will not be difficult. You want to determine what impact the illness has had on the individual and on the family.

The following questions will allow you to understand the impact of the condition on the person and on his or her family.

What disorder does the person have?

When was the person initially diagnosed?

What was the person's initial reaction to the diagnosis?

What was required for the person's adjustment to the condition?

How did the family react to the diagnosis?

How has the person's chronic condition changed the way that family members interact with each other?

What other changes have occurred in the family as a result of this person's condition?

What positive changes have occurred as a result of the condition?

What negative changes have occurred as a result of the condition?

How was the experience of living with a chronic illness different than what you imagined before you had the experience?

Answers

Fill in the Rest of the Story

I.   chronic
I.A.   negative; groups
I.B.   adaptation; caregivers; grief
II.   brain; age; lipoprotein
II.A.   sensory
II.B.   wander; support
III.   Type 2; blood glucose; dietary; exercise
III.A. insulin; glucagon; sugar (glucose); cardiovascular
III.B. lifetime; comply (adhere)
III.C. conceptualize (perceive); stress; compliance (adherence)
IV.   African; children
IV.A.   bronchial; allergic; cleanliness
IV.B.   triggers; weight
V.   human immunodeficiency virus; opportunistic
V.A.   decreased; living longer
V.B.   injection drug; mother; infant; heterosexual
V.C.   influenza; immune; opportunistic; AIDS
V.D.   sexual; male; male, injection; second; heterosexual contact; condom
V.E.   high-risk; needles; unprotected (unsafe)
VI.   good death
VI.A.   order (sequence); dying; relational
VI.B.   loss; grief; grieving; negative

Multiple Choice

1.	b	9.	b	16.	b	24.	a
2.	c	10.	a	17.	d	25.	c
3.	b	11.	b	18.	c	26.	c
4.	d	12.	b	19.	d	27.	c
5.	d	13.	d	20.	d	28.	c
6.	c	14.	c	21.	c	29.	a
7.	d	15.	c	22.	a	30.	b
8.	b			23.	b		

Matching

1.	e	2.	c	3.	g	4.	i	5.	f
6.	a	7.	d	8.	j	9.	b	10.	h

Good points to include in your essay answers:

1. A. Both types of diabetes mellitus have the psychological impact of living with an incurable disease and require lifestyle changes and self-care in order for these patients to survive and to avoid medical complications.
    1. Living with a chronic disease can produce denial, which can lead diabetics to ignore their condition and avoid proper self-care.
    2. Diabetics who accept their condition can be angry or resentful, which can also influence their self-care.
    B. Stress is a factor in blood glucose regulation for some diabetics.
    C. Patients' understanding of diabetes and their perception of symptoms affect their behavior, including what symptoms require a response and what response they choose.
    D. The lifestyle changes for diabetes management are a compliance problem that is especially difficult for children and adolescents.
    1. Feeling abnormal or left out of normal activities can be difficult for children and adolescents.
    2. Adhering to a complex regimen of diet, glucose testing, and insulin injections is a difficult regimen to manage.

2. A. The statement is not true because the drugs do not prevent and do not cure HIV infection.
    1. Drugs and medical treatment have made a difference in survival time for those infected with HIV.
    2. The modes of infection are behavioral, and the only way of slowing the spread of infection is behavioral interventions.
    B. Psychologists study behavior, the major mode of transmission of the virus.
    1. Psychologists devise interventions to change high-risk behaviors.
    2. Psychologists study the behavioral manifestations of HIV infection on the central nervous system.
    C. Psychologists also play an important role in providing health care for those with HIV.
    1. Psychologists offer counseling to those who are considering HIV testing to help them cope with the stress of deciding and learning about their HIV status.
    2. Psychologists offer counseling to those who are infected with HIV, helping them manage the distress of the diagnosis.
    3. Psychologists counsel those who are HIV infected so that they will not pass on their infection and so that they will adopt healthier lives.

CHAPTER 12
Smoking Tobacco

Learning Objectives

After studying Chapter 12, you should be able to

1. Explain how smoking affects the respiratory system.

2. Trace the history of smoking.

3. Describe the characteristics that differentiate smokers from nonsmokers.

4. Contrast the factors that relate to smoking initiation versus the factors that maintain the smoking habit.

5. Identify the risks associated with cigarette smoking.

6. Evaluate the risks for forms of tobacco use other than cigarette smoking.

7. Compare the risks of smoking to those of passive smoking.

8. Evaluate the effectiveness of interventions to deter smoking.

9. Explain what methods of quitting are more effective.

10. Discuss the consequences of quitting, identifying both negative and positive consequences.

Fill in the Rest of the Story

I. Smoking and the Respiratory System

The respiratory system functions to take _____ into the body and to

remove _____ _____.

A. Functioning of the Respiratory System

Air is taken into the body through the mouth or nose through contractions of the

_____. From the mouth or nose, it travels past the larynx, down the trachea

and _____ tubes, and into the lungs. Airborne particles such as smoke and

other pollutants easily enter the body through the _____ system, but the

body has several protective mechanisms, such as sneezing and _____ to

expel some of these dangerous particles. Respiratory disorders of most interest to health

psychologists are the chronic _____ respiratory diseases of bronchitis (inflammation of the bronchi) and _____, a chronic lung disease in which

scar tissue and mucus obstruct the respiratory passages.

B. What Components in Smoke Are Dangerous?

The principal drug in tobacco is _____, a stimulant drug that is

extremely toxic in large doses, although its harmful effects on smokers are hard to measure.

Other potentially dangerous byproducts include acrolein and formaldehyde, which belong to

a class of irritating compounds called _____, along with nitric oxide

and hydrocyanic acid.

II. A Brief History of Tobacco Use

Although Native Americans smoked tobacco before the voyages of Columbus, when the

early European explorers discovered tobacco, they quickly took to the smoking habit. However,

cigarettes did not gain popularity until the early years of the _____ century.

Until the decade of the _____, few people suspected that smoking presented health hazards,

and physicians often recommended smoking to their patients.

III. Choosing to Smoke

People who choose to smoke increase their risk of a variety of diseases, the most deadly of

which are _____ cancer, _____ disease, and

chronic _____ _____ disease.

A. Who Smokes and Who Does Not?

Currently, about _____% of the adults in the United States smoke, and this

percentage has _____ since the 1960s. Presently, (and for the first time

since records have been kept) there are more _____ smokers in the

United States than current smokers. In the past, men smoked at much higher rates than

women, but now _____ level is a better predictor of smoking than gender.

B. Why Do People Smoke?

Each year in the United States nearly _____ teenagers begin smoking,

and many believe that they can and will quit before they suffer from any of the dangers of smoking. People begin smoking for a variety of reasons, but most begin as

_____ when peer pressure is strong. Most young smokers believe that

they will not be smoking in a few more years. Other reasons for teenagers to begin smoking

include genetics and advertising. In addition, many teenage girls begin smoking as a means

of _____ control.

People may continue to smoke for several reasons. One reason is that smokers become

_____ to the drug nicotine. This view can explain why people continue to

smoke but fails to explain why people _____.

People who enjoy the taste and aroma of cigarettes continue to smoke because they are

being _____ reinforced for smoking, whereas others continue to smoke

because they experience painful withdrawal sensations when they try to

_____. Another reason why many people continue to smoke is that they

believe that the negative consequences of smoking apply to others but not to them; that is,

they have an _____ _____. Finally, many people, especially

_____ continue to smoke because they fear weight gain.

IV. Health Consequences of Tobacco Use

Cigarette smoking is the leading cause of preventable disease and death in the United

States, accounting for about _____ deaths a year, which is about 20% of all

deaths.

A. Cigarette Smoking

Smoking plays a role in the development of several cancers, especially

_____ cancer. In addition, smokers _____ their risk for

cardiovascular disease, and their risk for chronic lower _____ diseases

are sharply increased. Unlike CVD and cancer, deaths from lower respiratory diseases have

_____ dramatically during the past 25 years until it is now the

_____ leading cause of death in the United States

Compared with nonsmokers, smokers tend to have higher rates of diseases of the mouth. They are also more likely to be diagnosed with a _____ disorder such as depression or a substance abuse problem. They experience a variety of physical problems, and female smokers who are at elevated risk to deliver _____-_____-_____ babies.

B. Cigar and Pipe Smoking

Cigar and pipe smoking are neither as common nor as _____ as cigarette smoking, provided that these smokers do not inhale. Cigars and pipe smokers, however, experience elevated risk of _____ cancer and several other cancers (especially of the mouth, pharynx, esophagus, and larynx) as well as cardiovascular diseases.

C. Passive Smoking

Passive smoking, also called _____ tobacco smoke (ETS), is a risk for several diseases and disorders. People exposed to environmental tobacco smoke have only a slightly elevated _____ risk for lung cancer because the comparison group (lung cancer patients who have not been exposed to passive smoking) is quite _____. Thus, the relative risk of 1.2 or so means that very few nonsmokers develop lung cancer as a result of being exposed to passive smoking. Women married to smokers for 30 years or more show no greater number of these deaths than women married to nonsmokers.

Although the relative risk of passive smoking on heart disease is about the same as it is for lung cancer (1.2 to 1.3), environmental tobacco smoke claims far _____ victims from heart disease than from lung cancer. This situation exists because heart disease has a much higher prevalence than lung cancer.

Children less than two years old whose mothers smoke have a twofold risk of death from _____ _____ _____ syndrome (SIDS). In addition, infants face a number of other conditions, including _____, pneumonia,

asthma, lower respiratory tract illnesses, low birth weight, and childhood cancers.

D. Smokeless Tobacco

Use of smokeless tobacco rose sharply during the 1980s and 1990s among

_____ American teenage boys, who tend to believe that this form of

tobacco is safer than cigarette smoking. However, smokeless tobacco has been associated

with increased rates of _____ cancer and periodontal disease.

V. Interventions for Reducing Smoking Rates

Programs aimed at reducing smoking rates can be divided into two types: those that deter

people from beginning and those that encourage current smokers to _____.

A. Deterring Smoking

Most educational programs aimed at preventing young people from smoking have a

_____ success rate, but programs integrated into comprehensive health

_____ with booster sessions over years are more successful, especially when

embedded within _____-_____ anti-smoking campaigns.

B. Quitting Smoking

Although quitting is not easy, about _____% of U.S. adults have quit. Most people

who have quit smoking have done so _____ _____

_____. Nicotine replacement therapy, which comes in the form of nicotine

gum, spray, lozenges, inhalers, or _____is more effective in helping people

quit than a _____. Nicotine replacement therapy is often combined with

psychological approaches, including behavior _____, cognitive behavior

techniques, contracts, group therapy, social support, relaxation training, stress management,

and "booster" sessions. Smokers who have the support of family members and who believe

that they can quit; that is, those with high _____-_____

have higher quit rates than do smokers without these conditions. Women seem to have lower

quit rates than men, but this difference is at least partially explained by evidence showing that female smokers face more obstacles to quitting. In addition to gender, having strong

_____ support and a diagnosis of heart disease prompts quitting, whereas

heavy use of _____ makes quitting more difficult

C. Relapse Prevention

Many people who quit smoking (or other unhealthy behaviors) equate a single slip with

total _____. Nevertheless, relapse need not be permanent, and many

smokers continue in cycles of quitting and relapse until they quit permanently.

VI. Effects of Quitting

Quitting smoking is likely to bring about two health-related effects; better health and

_____ gain.

A. Quitting and Weight Gain

Several factors relate to quitting smoking and subsequent weight gain. First, most

smokers _____ some weight when they stop smoking, but the average

weight gain is modest, about _____ pounds. Men and women gain about the same

number of pounds. For most ex-smokers, much of the weight gain is

_____. Increased _____ _____ can

curtail weight gain, and cognitive behavior therapy can help change both physical activity

and eating habits.

B. Health Benefits of Quitting

By quitting smoking, both men and women can increase their _____

expectancy, quickly decrease their risk of _____ disease, and more slowly

decrease their risk for _____ cancer.

Multiple Choice Questions

_____ 1. Through the respiratory system, the body takes in oxygen and eliminates
   a. nitrogen.
   b. methane.
   c. carbon dioxide.
   d. nitrogen and carbon dioxide.

_____ 2. Anna coughs whenever she first inhales cigarette smoke. Anna should know that coughing
   a. is a probable sign of lung cancer.
   b. is nature's way of expelling irritants from the respiratory tract.
   c. draws oxygen more deeply into the lungs.
   d. is a certain symptom of bronchitis.

_____ 3. The percentage of adults in the United States who smoke is currently declining from the peak it reached
   a. during the Civil War.
   b. during the 1920s.
   c. during the 1960s.
   d. during the 1980s.

_____ 4. The current decline in smoking rates can be traced to
   a. the effectiveness of hypnosis in smoking cessation programs.
   b. the 1964 Surgeon General's report.
   c. the 1985 ban on depicting smoking in Hollywood movies.
   d. the failure of tobacco companies to achieve their goal of appearing as good corporate citizens.

_____ 5. The primary addictive drug in cigarettes is
   a. hydrocyanic acid.
   b. nitric oxide.
   c. acrolein.
   d. nicotine.

_____ 6. Currently, people who have the highest rate of smoking in the United States
   a. have a college education.
   b. are African American.
   c. are female.
   d. both a and b.
   e. none of the above.

_____ 7. Which factor has the strongest inverse relationship to smoking rates?
   a. age
   b. weight
   c. level of psychological well-being
   d. educational level

_____ 8. Each year in the United States about 438,000 people die of smoking-related causes; and each year, about _____ teenagers begin to smoke.
   a. 200,000
   b. 400,000
   c. 700,000
   d. 2 million

_____ 9. Most teenagers who begin smoking are familiar with the dangers of this practice, but they do not believe that they are in danger. Such a belief is known as
   a. the ostrich attitude.
   b. self-deceit.
   c. smoking blindness.
   d. an optimistic bias.

_____ 10. What is the best answer to the question of why people smoke?
   a. People smoke in order to have something to do with their hands.
   b. People smoke because it is a habit they cannot break.
   c. People smoke in order to lose weight.
   d. People smoke for a variety of reasons.

_____ 11. Palmer is 15 years old and has smoked a total of 200 cigarettes. If he tries to quit,
   a. he will be able to do so more easily than someone 25 years old.
   b. he will be able to do so with little difficulty.
   c. he will probably find it very difficult to quit.
   d. he will probably begin to drink or use other drugs.

_____ 12. Blanca smokes about 30 cigarettes a day. When she is NOT smoking, she is very much aware of this fact. Blanca is probably
   a. an addictive smoker.
   b. a weight conscious smoker.
   c. receiving some hidden reward for smoking.
   d. receiving negative punishment for smoking.

_____ 13. Sales of American tobacco companies are likely to remain strong because
   a. tobacco markets in Africa, Eastern Europe, and Asia are expanding.
   b. tobacco companies are now using subliminal advertising to motivate young people to begin smoking.
   c. former cigarette smokers are switching to cigars and pipes, which consume more tobacco than do cigarettes.
   d. more middle age and older adults are beginning to smoke.

_____ 14. Evidence that cigarette smoking is a greater risk than environmental pollution for lung cancer comes from studies that found
   a. an increase in lung cancer among nonsmokers.
   b. a relatively stable pattern of lung cancer among nonsmokers and an increase of lung cancer among smokers.
   c. a decrease in lung cancer among male smokers.
   d. a decrease in lung cancer among female smokers.

_____ 15. The explanation of smoking because of nicotine addiction
   a. is not supported by research evidence, which suggests that nicotine is a nonaddictive drug.
   b. fails to explain why some people are light smokers and some are heavy smokers.
   c. occurs in all heavy smokers but not in light smokers.
   d. does not apply to people who smoke pipes and cigars.

_____ 16. Tara wants to quit smoking, but every time she stops smoking she quickly experiences painful withdrawal symptoms. This suggests that Tara receives
   a. positive reinforcement for smoking.
   b. negative reinforcement for smoking.
   c. positive reinforcement for not smoking.
   d. negative reinforcement for not smoking.

_____ 17. Carla enjoys the aroma of her cigarettes. This suggests that Carla is receiving
   a. positive reinforcement for smoking.
   b. negative reinforcement for smoking.
   c. positive reinforcement for not smoking.
   d. negative reinforcement for not smoking.

_____ 18. Cigarette smoking leads to
   a. increased sexual potency among men.
   b. increased fertility among women.
   c. increased symptoms of depression.
   d. all of the above.

_____ 19. Compared with cigarette smokers, people who smoke only a pipe
   a. have a much lower risk of dying from lung cancer.
   b. have about the same risk of dying from lung cancer.
   c. have less than 1% the risk of dying from lung cancer.
   d. have a slightly increased risk of dying from lung cancer.

_____ 20. With regard to passive smoking and disease, research indicates that
   a. nonsmoking women married for 30 years to men who smoke triple their risk of breast cancer.
   b. more people die from passive smoking than from active smoking.
   c. passive smoking kills more people from cardiovascular disease than from lung cancer.
   d. passive smoking has no harmful effects on adults, that is, only children have been harmed by passive smoking.

_____ 21. The passive smokers who suffer the most adverse overall health effects from environmental tobacco smoke are
   a. young children of smoking parents.
   b. wives of smoking husbands.
   c. husbands of smoking wives.
   d. older parents of smoking children.

_____ 22. Which of these tactics is generally most effective in deterring young people from smoking?
   a. warnings on cigarette packs
   b. educational procedures
   c. threats of illness and early death
   d. extensive health education plus community campaign against smoking

_____ 23. Compared with quit rates from a placebo patch, the quit rates from a nicotine patch
   a. are about 10% lower.
   b. are about the same.
   c. are significantly higher.
   d. are more than 10 times higher.

_____ 24. Most smokers who have successfully quit
   a. did so through hypnosis.
   b. did so on their own.
   c. used the nicotine patch.
   d. used the nicotine inhaler.

_____ 25. Community-wide antismoking campaigns are not as powerful in getting smokers to quit as nicotine replacement or psychological interventions.
   a. This lack of success indicates that such campaigns are not worth continuing.
   b. These programs are more successful with long-time smokers than with teenagers, so they are successful for a few people.
   c. When the audience is targeted to a more specific group, the success rate increases and cost decreases.
   d. These programs affect many more people and thus prompt many people to quit.

_____ 26. Smoking cessation programs are more successful in getting people to _____ than to _____.
a. quit . . . prevent them from relapsing
b. smoke pipes or cigars . . . quit cigarettes
c. switch to alternatives to tobacco . . . quit smoking
d. attend a 12-step program . . . use nicotine replacement

_____ 27. Alma would like to quit smoking, but she is afraid of gaining weight. Research indicates that
a. her fears have no basis—most people who quit gain less than 5 pounds.
b. her fears have some basis, but women gain very little weight after quitting, whereas men gain over 15 pounds on the average.
c. her fears have some basis—both women and men average about an 11-pound gain after quitting.
d. her fears have some basis—she would be healthier staying at normal weight and continuing to smoke.

_____ 28. On average, if a man with no heart disease were to follow a diet of no more than 10% of calories from saturated fat, he would extend his life a matter of a few weeks. If the same man were to quit smoking, he would extend his life by
a. about the same length of time.
b. about 3 or 4 months.
c. about 3 or 4 years.
d. about 7 to 8 years.

_____ 29. Henrietta has been a light smoker for about 20 years. If she quits smoking, her mortality risk will
a. be unaffected.
b. return to that of a nonsmoker in about 2 to 3 years.
c. return to that of a nonsmoker in about 16 years.
d. increase due to a change in lifestyle.

Key Terms

Define each of the following:

aldehydes —

bronchitis —

emphysema —

ETS —

formaldehyde —

muscocillary escalator —

nicotine —

nicotine replacement therapy —

passive smoking —

Matching

Match the following:

1. educational level

2. attention to cigarette advertising

3. byproducts of tobacco smoke

4. nicotine

5. relief from withdrawal symptoms

6. emphysema

7. smokers' failure to acknowledge their risk of heart disease

8. male smokers have a 23.3 relative risk for

9. passive smoking

10. increased risk for oral cancer

a. increases teenagers' risk for smoking

b. negative reinforcement

c. scar tissue and mucus obstruct the respiratory tract

d. best predictor of smoking status

e. optimistic bias

f. lung cancer

g. environmental tobacco smoke

h. smokeless tobacco

i. addictive component in tobacco

j. acrolein, formaldehyde, and hydrocyanic acid

1. _____   2. _____   3. _____   4. _____   5. _____

6. _____   7. _____   8. _____   9. _____   10. _____

How Smoking Affects the Lungs

Fill in the missing information concerning how smoking damages the lungs and respiratory function.

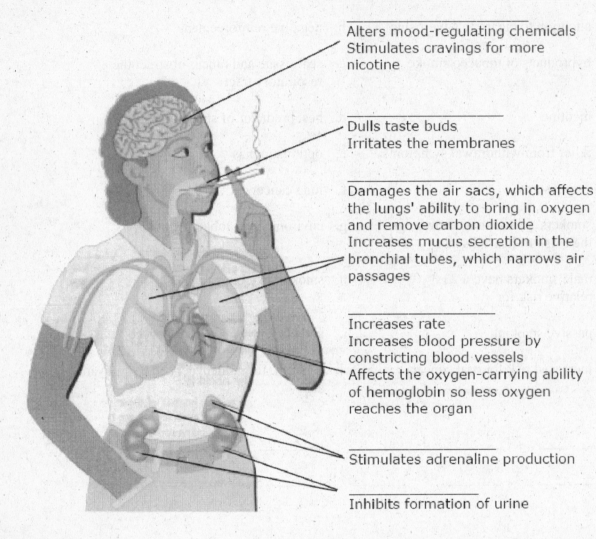

_____
Alters mood-regulating chemicals
Stimulates cravings for more
nicotine

_____
Dulls taste buds
Irritates the membranes

_____
Damages the air sacs, which affects
the lungs' ability to bring in oxygen
and remove carbon dioxide
Increases mucus secretion in the
bronchial tubes, which narrows air
passages

_____
Increases rate
Increases blood pressure by
constricting blood vessels
Affects the oxygen-carrying ability
of hemoglobin so less oxygen
reaches the organ

_____
Stimulates adrenaline production

_____
Inhibits formation of urine

Essay Questions

1. Evaluate the dangers of passive smoking, explaining who is at risk and what type of risk.

2. What advantages do the nicotine replacement therapies have over other methods of quitting?

Let's Get Personal— Risk from Smoke Exposure

Most college students do not smoke, thus avoiding the risks associated with cigarettes. A more common smoking-related risk is exposure to passive smoke, and many people are exposed under a variety of circumstances. Evaluate the degree of risk for exposure to various types of smoke, and examine your smoking habits and exposure in the various categories. Compared with nonsmokers, what is the risk of:

Lung cancer for smokers?

Lung cancer for nonsmoking spouses of smokers?

Lung cancer for nonsmokers who work with smokers?

Heart disease for smokers?

Heart disease for nonsmoking spouses of smokers?

Answers

Fill in the Rest of the Story

I.   oxygen; carbon dioxide

I.A.   diaphragm; bronchial; respiratory; coughing; lower; emphysema

I.B.   nicotine; aldehydes

II.   20th; 1960s

III.   lung; cardiovascular; lower respiratory

III.A. 21; declined; former; education

III.B   700,000; teenagers (adolescents); weight; addicted; begin; positively; quit; optimistic bias; women

IV   438,000

IV.A.   lung; increase; respiratory; increased; third; psychiatric, low-birth-weight

IV.B.   deadly (dangerous); lung

IV.C.   environmental; absolute; small; more; sudden infant death; bronchitis

IV.D.   European; oral

V.   quit

V.A.   low; education; community-wide

V.B.   23; on their own; patches; placebo; modification; self-efficacy; social; alcohol

V.C.   relapse

VI.   weight

VI.A.   gain; 11; temporary; physical activity

VI.B.   life; heart (cardiovascular); lung

Multiple Choice Answers

1.	c	9.	d	16.	b	23.	c
2.	b	10.	d	17.	a	24.	b
3.	c	11.	c	18.	c	25.	d
4.	b	12.	a	19.	a	26.	a
5.	d	13.	a	20.	c	27.	c
6.	e	14.	b	21.	a	28.	d
7.	d	15.	b	22.	d	29.	c
8.	c						

Matching

1.	d	2.	a	3.	j	4.	i	5.	b
6.	c	7.	e	8.	f	9.	g	10.	h

Good points to include in your essay answers:

1. A. Passive smoking or environmental tobacco smoke (ETS) is not as much of a risk as smoking cigarettes.
   B. For adults, ETS is irritating and annoying but poses relatively minor health risks.
      1. The risk of lung cancer is slightly elevated by passive smoking.
      2. The risk of heart disease is elevated by ETS, which presents a more widespread risk than that from lung cancer.
   C. ETS is more of a risk for children, increasing the risk of several problems.
      1. Infants who live with smokers are at increased risk of respiratory diseases and sudden infant death syndrome.
      2. Smoking is a danger for the unborn, being associated with low birth weight.
      3. The dangers decrease after children pass age 2 years.

2. A. Nicotine replacement therapy has become a popular treatment for smoking.
      1. Nicotine replacement therapy has several forms, including nicotine chewing gum, patches, inhalers, lozenges, and sprays.
      2. Nicotine replacement is sometimes used as the sole treatment, but it is sometimes combined with other treatment components in a multimodal program.
      3. Nicotine gum, patches, inhalers, spray, and lozenges are significantly more effective than placebo treatment.
   B. A combination of behavioral therapy and nicotine replacement is more effective than nicotine replacement therapy alone.

CHAPTER 13
Using Alcohol and Other Drugs

Learning Objectives

After studying Chapter 13, you should be able to

1. Trace the history of alcohol consumption in Europe and the United States.

2. Describe current patterns of drinking.

3. Describe the physical and behavioral effects of alcohol consumption.

4. Evaluate the direct and indirect effects of drinking.

5. Analyze the risks and benefits of drinking.

6. Compare and evaluate the theories of drinking, considering their adequacy to explain problem and nonproblem drinking.

7. Compare the success of treatments for problem drinking oriented toward abstinence and those with controlled drinking as the goal.

8. Describe the problem of relapse for both alcohol and drug abuse treatment.

9. Distinguish among drug use, drug misuse, and drug abuse.

10. Evaluate the health effects and the social effects of drug abuse.

11. Contrast drug use treatment with treatment for alcohol abuse.

Fill in the Rest of the Story

I. Alcohol Consumption—Yesterday and Today

The use of alcohol is as old as civilization (and possibly older). The consumption of alcohol brings both problems and benefits.

A. A Brief History of Alcohol Consumption

In colonial America, drinking was much more common than it is today, partially because _____ and milk were not always purified. The Puritans objected to _____ but not to drinking. Alcohol consumption in the United States _____ sharply after 1830 and rose after the _____ _____ was repealed in 1934 by the 21st Amendment.

B. The Prevalence of Alcohol Consumption Today

About _____ _____ of the adults in the United States are classified as current drinkers (defined as having at least one drink in the past year), about 20% engage in _____ drinking (five or more drinks on the same occasion at least once per month), and about 5% are _____ drinkers (14 or more drinks per week for men or 7 per week for women). Younger people drink more than older people, and they are more likely to _____ drink. Of the various ethnic groups in the United States, _____ Americans have the highest rates of alcohol consumption; _____ Americans the highest binge drinking rates. Drinking is more common among people with _____ levels of education.

II. The Effects of Alcohol

The specific alcohol used in beverages, which is a poison and can cause sudden death when consumed in large quantities, is called _____. Alcohol is one of the drugs that can lead to a situation in which progressively more of the drug is required to produce a constant effect. In other words, alcohol can produce _____. It can also produce dependence and _____ symptoms in the form of delirium tremens. The combination of dependence and withdrawal symptoms is what some people refer to as _____.

A. Hazards of Alcohol

Alcohol produces a variety of hazards, both direct and indirect. One direct hazard is the accumulation of fat in the liver, which may eventually lead to _____, a major cause of death among people addicted to alcohol. Prolonged, heavy drinking may also cause neurological damage, and _____ syndrome, which results in severe memory loss and cognitive dysfunction. Heavy drinkers may also have a slight increase in risks for cancer of the esophagus, stomach, and liver. In large doses, alcohol can impair the heart's ability to function properly, lead to hypertension, and cause stroke.

Women who drink excessively during pregnancy sometimes give birth to an infant with

_____ _____ syndrome, a disorder that includes growth

deficiencies, central nervous system dysfunction, and mental retardation. Indirect and

harmful consequences of alcohol include diminished coordination and judgment, which

greatly increase the risk of _____ _____.

Alcohol is involved in about two thirds of the _____ in the United States

and about _____% of fatal motor vehicle crashes.

B. Benefits of Alcohol

Several studies have reported a J-shaped relationship between alcohol consumption and

health, with nondrinkers and heavy drinkers at a(n) _____ risk. Most of

the benefits of light and moderate drinking come from reduced _____

disease, which offsets increased risk from other sources of mortality. The decrease in CHD

mortality seems to be due to increases in _____-_____

lipoprotein. Moderate consumption of alcohol lowers the rates of ulcers, gallstones, Type

_____ diabetes, and Alzheimer's disease.

III. Why Do People Drink?

Several models have been suggested to explain why people drink. Historically, the

_____ model has had the greatest influence on therapies for alcohol

addiction.

A. The Disease Model

During the past 50 years, the medical profession has advocated a

_____ model of alcoholism. Because alcoholism tends to run in

families, a _____ component has been part of the disease model, but

research indicates that environmental influences also contribute. One model, which is more

flexible than the traditional disease model, emphasizes _____ control

instead of loss of control or the inability to abstain. According to this model—called the

_____ _____ model, seven components

233

make up a syndrome of drinking-related behaviors: (1) narrowing of drinking repertoire,

(2) salience of _____-seeking behavior, (3) increased

_____, (4) withdrawal symptoms, (5) avoidance of withdrawal by more

_____ (6) subjective awareness of the need to drink, and (7)

reinstatement of _____ after abstinence.

Disease models offer a reasonable explanation for why some people drink too much,

but they are less successful in giving reasons why people _____ to drink. Some

research suggests that craving for alcohol results from drinkers'

_____ of alcohol's effects, rather than from physical properties of

alcohol.

B. Cognitive-Physiological Theories

Several alternatives to the disease model emphasize the combination of physiological

and _____ changes that occur with alcohol use. The tension reduction

hypothesis assumes that people drink as a means of coping with _____.

Alcohol is a _____ drug, so it is capable of producing physiological

relaxation and slowed reactions. However, alcohol's effects are not consistent, which has

led to a reformulation of the tension reduction model called the stress-response-dampening

effect. This model showed that alcohol _____ the strength of

responses to stress. The notion that alcohol creates effects on social behaviors that produce

a kind of shortsightedness while blocking out insightful cognitive processing is called

_____ _____.

C. The Social Learning Model

Many psychologists accept social learning theory, which suggests that drinking

behavior is _____; that is, it is acquired through positive or

negative _____ and by observing others; that is, through

_____. Social learning theory assumes that people can also learn to abstain or to drink in moderation. Thus the goal of treatment might be either abstinence or

_____ drinking.

IV. Changing Problem Drinking

Gender is a strong predictor of who will seek treatment for alcoholism, with

_____ far out-numbering _____.

A. Change without Therapy

Many people quit drinking without going into a treatment program. The term

_____ _____ applies to disease cures that occur

without treatment, but for those who do not consider problem drinking a disease, this term

is not appropriate. The term _____ change may be more accurate, but

this too may be misleading because most problems drinkers who quit without formal

treatment have had the help of family and friends.

B. Treatments Oriented toward Abstinence

All treatment programs have _____ as their immediate goal,

although some include controlled drinking as an ultimate goal. Probably the most common

treatment approach in the United States, and one that is often included as an adjunct to

other abstinence programs is _____ _____. The

anonymity component makes research difficult, but this program produces a high

_____ rate. AA can help some problem drinkers but is not well suited to

many people.

Psychotherapy programs are successful in getting most heavy drinkers to reduce their

consumption to some extent, but only about _____% of problem drinkers are abstinent

after one year. Some alcohol treatment programs include _____

(Antabuse) or other drugs that interact with alcohol to produce unpleasant effects. This

approach is called _____ therapy, which is based on the notion that

drinking will become unpleasant because of the association with unpleasant consequences.

The major problem with this type of therapy is _____; patients are not eager to take a drug that will make them sick if they drink alcohol. Other drugs may be more effective in controlling cravings and preventing relapse.

C. Controlled Drinking

Since the 1960s, therapists have observed that a small percentage of recovered alcoholics were able drink in a _____ fashion, even in programs aimed at abstinence. In addition, many former problem drinkers have learned to control consumption on their own. Nevertheless, controlled drinking remains a controversial issue and is rarely a treatment goal in the _____ _____, but controlled drinking is a more common goal in the United Kingdom and Australia. Controlled drinking is not an acceptable goal for all problem drinkers, especially for _____ people with a long history of problem drinking.

D. The Problem of Relapse

Relapse rates for alcohol treatment are almost identical to those for drug abuse or _____. Most relapse training programs are aimed at changing _____ so that the addict comes to believe that one slip does *not* equal total relapse.

V. Other Drugs

In the United States, illicit drugs have created more _____ problems than health problems.

A. Health Effects

Potential health hazards are not limited to illicit drugs; _____ drugs can also pose a risk. Included in the list of legal drugs are _____ that induce relaxation by lowering the activity of the brain and even slowing metabolic rate. Sedative drugs include tranquilizers and alcohol, which have additive effects that make them dangerous when taken in combination or in large amounts. Barbiturates are synthetic drugs used medically to induce _____ but used recreationally to induce euphoria or intoxication. Morphine, heroin, and other _____ drugs have been used medically to relieve pain, but they produce both tolerance and dependence after only a short time.

Drugs that produce alertness, reduce feelings of fatigue, elevate mood, and decrease

appetite include amphetamines, which are classified as _____

drugs. Cocaine acts as a stimulant to the _____ system, and the

strength and duration of its action depend on both dose and mode of administration.

MDMA ("_____") is a derivative of methamphetamine but used for

its mild hallucinogenic effects, including feelings of peace and well being. The most

commonly used illegal drug in the United States is _____, which has

also been used medically to prevent the vomiting associated with chemotherapy and to treat

the eye disease called _____. Some people use anabolic steroids to

increase _____ bulk or to improve appearance, but medically,

steroids are used to reduce inflammation and to control some allergic reactions.

B. Drug Misuse and Abuse

All psychoactive drugs, including those used primarily for _____

purposes, are potentially dangerous. When people take drugs in an inappropriate but not

health-threatening manner, they _____ that drug; they

_____ a drug when their consumption is frequent, heavy, and harmful to their

health.

C. Treatment for Drug Abuse

Treatment for illegal drug abuse is similar to the treatment for _____

abuse. The immediate goal for both is _____. As with alcohol

treatments, programs for drug abuse suffer from high _____ rates.

D. Preventing and Controlling Drug Use

Drug prevention programs that rely on scare tactics, moral training, factual

information about drug risks, and boosting self-esteem generally have

_____ success rates, but school programs that teach social skills are

somewhat more successful.

Multiple Choice Questions

_____ 1. A man who drinks one to three drinks a day is considered a
   a. light drinker.
   b. light to moderate drinker.
   c. heavy drinker.
   d. binge drinker.

_____ 2. In the United States, the peak consumption of alcohol occurred
   a. around 1820 to 1830.
   b. during the Civil War.
   c. during Prohibition.
   d. during the 1960s
   e. during the early 1990s.

_____ 3. In the United States
   a. about 90% of the people drink alcohol, about 40% are binge drinkers, and about 20% are heavy drinkers.
   b. about 50% of the people drink alcohol, and about half of these abuse alcohol.
   c. about two thirds of the population are drinkers, 20% are binge drinkers, and 5% are heavy drinkers.
   d. about one third of the population abuse alcohol to the point that it interferes with their health.

_____ 4. Which group has the highest rate of alcohol consumption in the United States?
   a. young and middle-aged adults
   b. women
   c. older adults
   d. young adolescents

_____ 5. Which of these statements is true?
   a. Drinking rates are currently going up.
   b. Women drink more than men.
   c. The rate of drinking has declined over the past 20 years.
   d. African Americans drink more than Asian Americans.
   e. All of the above are true.

_____ 6. Seymour finds himself drinking more in order to maintain the same effects of alcohol. The term that best describes Seymour's condition is
   a. tolerance.
   b. withdrawal.
   c. physical dependence.
   d. psychological dependence.

_____ 7. Celeste has a long history of heavy drinking. She finds herself needing to have a drink in order to go to work, to talk to her sister, to sleep, or to do about anything else. The term that best describes Celeste's condition is
   a. tolerance.
   b. dependence.
   c. withdrawal.
   d. psychological tolerance.

_____ 8. Benita has recently quit drinking after years of alcohol abuse. Now she finds herself restless, irritable, agitated, and shaky. Benita is experiencing
   a. tolerance.
   b. psychological dependence.
   c. physiological dependence.
   d. withdrawal symptoms.

_____ 9. Drugs that produce dependence and that, when discontinued, result in withdrawal symptoms are called
   a. addictive drugs.
   b. psychoactive drugs.
   c. tolerance drugs.
   d. illicit drugs.

_____ 10. Claude has a long history of excessive and chronic alcohol abuse and now has confusion, poor memory for recent events, and severe disorientation. Claude is exhibiting symptoms of
   a. aldehyde dehydrogenase psychosis.
   b. psychological withdrawal.
   c. delirium tremens.
   d. Korsakoff syndrome.

_____ 11. Heavy consumption of alcohol generally
   a. decreases a woman's fertility.
   b. increases a woman's fertility.
   c. has no effect on a woman's fertility.
   d. leads to higher birth weight of the baby.
   e. both b and d.

_____12. Which of the following is an indirect effect of alcohol?
   a. increased high-density lipoprotein cholesterol
   b. increased risk of cirrhosis of the liver
   c. increased risk of unintentional injuries
   d. increased risk of heart disease

_____13. Research on the relationship between alcohol consumption and death rate shows
   a. a J-shaped or U-shaped relationship.
   b. a W-shaped relationship.
   c. a direct and dose-response relationship between level of drinking and chances of mortality.
   d. an inverse relationship between level of drinking and chances of mortality.

_____14. The health benefits of moderate drinking apply to
   a. men but not to women.
   b. young adults but not to older adults.
   c. African Americans but not to European Americans.
   d. older adults but not to middle-aged or young adults.
   e. middle-aged adults but not to young adults.

_____15. Research shows that alcohol may confer some protection against heart disease because it
   a. lowers low-density lipoprotein.
   b. raises low-density lipoprotein.
   c. lowers high-density lipoprotein.
   d. raises high-density lipoprotein.

_____16. Which of these statements most accurately describes the relationship between consumption of alcohol and heart disease?
   a. Light to moderate daily drinking raises HDL, and thus lowers the risk of heart disease.
   b. Binge drinking raises HDL more than daily drinking.
   c. Alcohol greatly increases the risk of heart disease.
   d. Two or three drinks of a day raises LDL, and thus raises the risk of heart disease.

_____17. The disease model of alcohol consumption has been
   a. embraced by most psychologists for the past 50 years.
   b. embraced by the U.S. medical community for the past 50 years.
   c. abandoned by the majority of those who provide treatment for problem drinking.
   d. both a and b.

_____18. A key concept of the disease model is
   a. a genetic predisposition to drink alcohol.
   b. impaired control, that is, the inability to stop drinking once drinking begins.
   c. a subjective awareness of the need to drink.
   d. loss of control, that is, the inability to abstain from alcohol.

_____19. Using the balanced placebo design, Marlatt and his colleagues found
    a. that alcoholics can be divided into three distinct groups.
    b. support for the tension reduction hypothesis.
    c. that intoxication can be more dangerous than had been previously observed.
    d. that the intoxication experienced from light to moderate drinking is strongly affected by expectancy.

_____20. Which of these concepts is NOT part of the alcohol dependency syndrome?
    a. inability to abstain
    b. narrowing of drinking repertoire
    c. salience of drinking behavior
    d. subjective awareness of the compulsion to drink

_____21. For many people, consumption of alcohol impairs their view of reality and changes the way they think about self, stress, and social anxiety. This describes
    a. the stress-response-dampening effect.
    b. gamma alcoholism.
    c. delta alcoholism.
    d. alcohol myopia.

_____22. The social learning model of drinking includes these terms:
    a. loss of control, inability to abstain, and disease.
    b. coping, modeling, and negative reinforcement.
    c. stress-response-dampening effect and delta alcoholic.
    d. increased tissue tolerance and adaptive cell metabolism.

_____23. People who drink in order to avoid the aversive consequences of withdrawal are demonstrating
    a. alcohol myopia.
    b. positive reinforcement.
    c. negative reinforcement.
    d. the balanced placebo effect.

_____24. Another term for quitting drinking without the aid of therapy is
    a. assisted change.
    b. stress-response dampening effect.
    c. spontaneous remission.
    d. disulfiram.

_____25. Alcohol abusers who are MOST likely to be successful at controlled drinking are
    a. people whose drinking problems are short-term and who have no physical damage from alcohol.
    b. older, married people who have at least a 40-year history of heavy drinking.
    c. people who have adopted the philosophy of Alcoholics Anonymous.
    d. people who have tried a variety of treatment approaches and who believe that they are physically dependent on alcohol.

_____26. One year after the end of treatment, about 35% of people completing a treatment program for _____ will still be abstinent.
    a. alcohol abuse
    b. opiate abuse
    c. smoking
    d. any of the above

_____27. Drugs that change the brain's chemistry, have side effects, and change perception
    a. are all regulated by the FDA.
    b. are specifically excluded from FDA regulation.
    c. are called sedatives.
    d. have crossed the blood-brain barrier.

_____28. Which of these drugs can produce both tolerance and dependence as quickly as 24 hours?
    a. opiates
    b. anabolic steroids
    c. benzodiazepines
    d. all of the above

_____29. The combination of cocaine and alcohol
    a. cancel the effects of each other, posing less danger than either taken separately.
    b. produces cocaethylene, a potentially deadly chemical, making the combination more dangerous than either separately.
    c. accounts for approximately 50% of the cases of people admitted to hospital emergency rooms.
    d. both b and c.

_____30. The Food and Drug Administration classifies marijuana as a Schedule I drug, which means that the FDA considers marijuana to
    a. be low in abuse potential, with no accepted medical use.
    b. be high in abuse potential, with some accepted medical use.
    c. be high in abuse potential, with no accepted medical use.
    d. to have no abuse potential, with some accepted medical use.

Key Terms

Define each of the following:

alcohol myopia —

anabolic steroids —

cirrhosis —

delirium tremens —

dependence —

fetal alcohol syndrome —

Korsakoff syndrome —

sedatives —

tolerance —

withdrawal —

Matching

Match the following:

1. marijuana

    a. demonstrates that expectancy influences drinkers

2. balanced placebo design

    b. withdrawal symptoms occur when a person discontinues the drug

3. drunken excess, self-inflation, and drunken relief

    c. the disease model of alcoholism

4. E. M. Jellinek

    d. unassisted quitting

5. tolerance

    e. return to nonproblem drinking by problem drinkers

6. dependence

    f. progressively more of the drug is required to produce the same effect

7. cirrhosis of the liver

    g. most frequently used illicit drug

8. spontaneous remission

    h. alcohol myopia

9. controlled drinking

    i. frequently used legal drug

10. ethanol

    j. risk associated with heavy drinking

1. _____ 2. _____ 3. _____ 4. _____ 5. _____

6. _____ 7. _____ 8. _____ 9. _____ 10. _____

The Balanced Placebo and Alcohol Expectancy Effects

The balanced placebo design has been important in separating expectancy effects from the pharmacological effects of alcohol. Demonstrate your understanding of this design by filling in the missing information from this figure of the balanced placebo design.

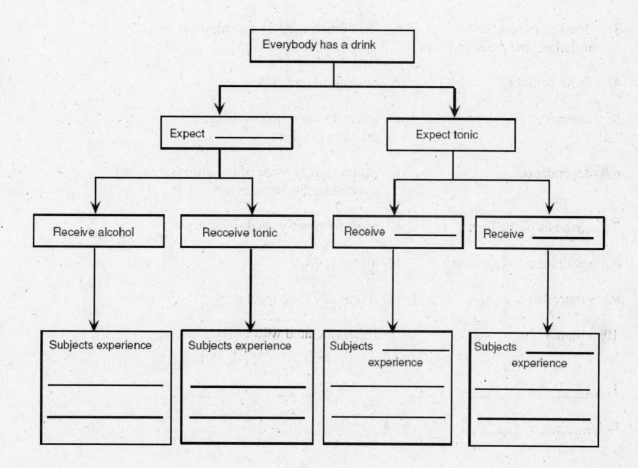

Essay Questions

1. Evaluate the statement, "There is both good news and bad news for people who drink."

2. Two 18-year-old high school seniors grew up in the same neighborhood. One young woman drinks, and the other does not. Using the social learning model, explain the difference.

Let's Get Personal—
How Do You Drink?

Drinking alcohol is a common practice for college students, and some college activities are oriented around drinking. College students, however, make a variety of choices concerning their intake of alcohol, with some choosing to abstain, some choosing light or moderate drinking, and others choosing binge or heavy drinking. What are your drinking habits? Examine your drinking pattern by answering these questions:

Do you drink alcohol?

Under what circumstances do you drink—at parties, when you go out, with meals at restaurants, with meals at home, after school or work, or some combination of these circumstances?

On how many days during the past month did you have anything to drink?

Was there one or more occasion during the past year on which you had five or more drinks?

When was the last time that you were intoxicated?

Regardless of your choices, your drinking habits have health implications. If you do not drink, you do not experience the risks associated with increased chances for unintentional injuries, but neither do you experience the potential cardiovascular and other health benefits. If you are a light or moderate drinker, you may receive benefits from your drinking patterns, but you also experience risks resulting from increased chances for unintentional injuries. The benefits may outweigh the risks, but drinking always carries some risk. If you drink heavily or in binges, you probably raise your risks for unintentional injury and liver damage more than you lower your cardiovascular and other health risks.

If your drinking does not conform to the pattern that confers benefits, what would you need to do to drink at that level? Is this a change you want to make?

Answers

Fill in the Rest of the Story

I.A.   water; drunkenness; dropped; 18th Amendment
I.B.   two thirds; binge; heavy; binge; European; Native; higher
II.   ethanol; tolerance; withdrawal; addiction
II.A. cirrhosis; Korsakoff; fetal alcohol; unintentional injuries; homicides; 30
II.B. increased (elevated); cardiovascular (heart); high-density; 2
III.   disease (medical)
III.A. disease; genetic; impaired; alcohol dependency; drink; tolerance; drinking; drinking (dependence); begin; expectations
III.B. cognitive; tension (stress); sedative (depressant); decreases; alcohol myopia
III.C. learned; reinforcement; modeling (observation); controlled
IV.   men; women
IV.A. spontaneous remission; unassisted
IV.B. abstinence; Alcoholics Anonymous; dropout; 25; disulfiram; aversion; compliance (adherence)
IV.C. controlled; United States; older
IV.D. smoking; cognitions (beliefs or perceptions)
V.   social
V.A.   legal (prescription); sedatives; sleep; opiate; stimulant; nervous; Ecstasy: marijuana; glaucoma; muscle (strength)
V.B.   medical; misuse; abuse
V.C.   alcohol; abstinence; relapse (dropout)
V.D.   low (limited)

Multiple Choice

1. b	9. a	16. a	24. c
2. a	10. d	17. b	25. a
3. c	11. a	18. d	26. d
4. a	12. c	19. d	27. d
5. c	13. a	20. a	28. a
6. a	14. e	21. d	29. b
7. b	15. d	22. b	30. c
8. d		23. c	

Matching

1. g	2. a	3. h	4. c	5. f
6. b	7. j	8. d	9. e	10. i

Good points to include in your essay answers:

1. A. The benefits outweigh the hazards for some patterns of drinking, whereas the hazards are more prominent for other patterns of drinking.
    B. Heavy drinking is a greater risk than benefit.
        1. People who drink heavily on a daily basis are more likely to experience the direct effects of alcohol—liver damage, Korsakoff syndrome, and fetal alcohol syndrome.
        2. Those who binge drink are at risk from the indirect effects of alcohol, including a variety of unintentional injuries, suicide, and homicide.
    C. Light and moderate drinking can bring greater benefits than risks.
        1. The risks of drinking still apply to these people, but the benefits can outweigh the risks.
        2. The main benefits come from lowered cardiovascular mortality, but health benefits include lowered risk of several other diseases.
        3. The benefits of light and moderate drinking apply to middle-aged and older adults but not to younger people.

2. A. The social learning model conceptualizes drinking as learned behavior, similar to other learned behaviors.
        1. People who drink must find reinforcement in drinking or some stimuli associated with it, or they would not drink.
        2. People who do not drink find more aversive than positive consequences in drinking, leading them to avoid drinking.
    B. For the young woman who drinks, the social learning model explains her drinking in terms of a greater balance of positive than aversive consequences. Many possibilities exist or combine to make her a drinker.
        1. She may have friends who encourage her drinking.
        2. She may enjoy going to places where drinking is the expected norm.
        3. She may like the taste of alcohol or the feeling of being intoxicated.
        4. She may be trying to cultivate an image that is consistent with drinking.
    C. For the young woman who does not drink, the social learning model explains that behavior in terms of a greater balance of negative than positive consequences associated with drinking.
        1. She may have negative physical reactions to alcohol, similar to the reaction that some Asians experience.
        2. She may not like the taste of alcohol.
        3. She may not like the feeling of intoxication.
        4. She may believe that drinking is wrong for moral or religious reasons.
        5. She may have friends or family whom she wishes to please who disapprove of drinking.

CHAPTER 14
Eating and Weight

Learning Objectives

After studying Chapter 14, you should be able to

1. Describe the function of the digestive system.

2. Analyze the factors that contribute to weight maintenance.

3. Discuss the evidence that supports and fails to support the two leading models of weight regulation.

4. Define obesity and discuss its effect on health.

5. Discuss the advantages and disadvantages of dieting.

6. Evaluate the various approaches to losing weight, considering both safety and effectiveness.

7. Contrast the risk factors and symptoms for anorexia and bulimia.

8. Compare treatment approaches and effectiveness for anorexia and bulimia.

9. Compare and contrast bulimia and binge eating, including both symptoms and characteristics of those with each disorder.

Fill in the Rest of the Story

I.   The Digestive System

The digestive system begins in the _____, where food is ground into small

particles and mixed with saliva from the salivary glands. After swallowing, food is propelled

through the esophagus and into the stomach by a process called _____.

Absorption of nutrients does not occur until food reaches the _____

_____. Bile salts produced in the _____ and stored in the gall

bladder break down fat molecules. Vitamins are manufactured and absorbed in the

_____ _____, and there the fluid volume of the mixture

is decreased.

II. Factors in Weight Maintenance

The weight equation consists of three factors: calories eaten, calories used in basal

metabolism, and calories expended through _____ _____.

Several hormones are also important to the long-term and short-term regulation of eating.

_____ levels fall when body fat decreases, sending a signal to eat. The brain contains

receptors for this hormone, especially in the _____. The hormone

_____ provides a short-term regulation of eating; the levels of this hormone rise

before and fall after meals. Another hormone, _____ (CCK) is related to

feelings of satiation.

A. Experimental Starvation

A study by Ancel Keys and his associates on experimental starvation indicated that the

body slows _____ to adjust for caloric restriction. Many of the volunteers

in Key's study had difficulty _____ weight, and they experienced

irritability, increased aggression, increased apathy as well as loss of

_____ interest and lethargy as a result of the food restriction. When

these men were permitted to eat as much as they wanted, most regained their lost weight

and many remained _____ with food and regained more weight than

they had lost.

B. Experimental Overeating

A study by Ethan Allen Sims and his associates on overfeeding showed that prison

volunteers found overeating _____ and weight gain increasingly

_____.

III. Overeating and Obesity

Because individual differences in metabolism allow some people to burn

_____ faster than others, overeating and _____ are not perfectly

related. However, overweight people usually eat more than normal weight people.

A. What Is Obesity?

Determining obesity is not easy, either by definition or by measurement techniques. A good definition should be percent of _____ _____, but this number is difficult to assess. The skinfold and water immersion techniques are more accurate in determining fat but are more awkward to use, and body imaging techniques are expensive. The _____ _____ index has been used more recently by researchers to determine distribution of weight. Standards for obesity have changed throughout history. Currently in the United States, thinness is valued, but _____ has increased dramatically during the past 20 years. Asian American women have the _____ rate of obesity, whereas _____ American women and Hispanic American _____ have the highest rates. Obesity is also increasing in nations around the world.

B. Why Are Some People Obese?

Several models have attempted to explain obesity, including the _____ model, which holds that weight is regulated by a type of internal thermostat that makes fluctuations in either direction difficult. However, people's weights vary, and researchers have established that a _____ component influences body weight and fat distribution. An alternative to the setpoint model, the _____ _____ model, assumes that positive reinforcement plays an important role in eating and weight maintenance. Thus, people may overeat for a variety of reasons, including food preferences, cultural influences on eating and body composition, and availability of _____.

C. How Unhealthy Is Obesity?

The question of obesity's effect on health depends on the method of measuring obesity, degree of obesity, and _____ of weight. The increased health risks of obesity are largest for _____ disease and diabetes. Fat around the _____ is more of a risk than fat on the

_____. After age _____, being overweight is no longer related to the

development of cardiovascular disease.

IV. Dieting

The increase in the number of people who are _____ or obese during the

1990s had led to an increased concern with dieting. Advertisements for "miracle" diets are

usually _____ because dieting must include eating fewer calories. People often

make unwise choices in dieting, which has become more widespread. Dieting is especially

common among _____ and women, who tend to adhere to a body ideal of

thinness.

A. Approaches to Losing Weight

Low-carbohydrate diets high in fat tend to be popular because they do not restrict the

amount of _____ and fat, but people have trouble staying on these diets.

Single-food diets, including liquid diets lead to weight loss due to greatly reduced

_____ as people become progressively bored with the single food.

Behavior modification programs for weight control attempt to

_____ healthy eating patterns and often included diet diaries, self-

rewards, and penalties for cheating.

One component of many diet programs is _____ because it speeds

body metabolism, builds muscle, and improves the ratio of muscle to fat. Diet pills and

surgery are _____ treatments that can produce weight loss but also

present health risks. Similar to treatment for smoking, problem drinking, and drug use, a

major problem for weight loss programs is _____, because a majority

of people who lose weight on any type of diet program will regain the lost weight.

B. Is Dieting a Good Choice?

Some experts recommend against dieting and counsel overweight people to stop

overeating and _____ regularly. Periodic dieting may be a poor choice for people over the age of _____ and normal-weight people. For many people who are

moderately overweight, maintaining a healthy lifestyle is a better choice than

_____.

V. Eating Disorders

Both anorexia nervosa and _____ begin as attempts to control weight,

and both may eventually produce dangerous physical effects. Binge eating is a contributor to

obesity.

A. Anorexia Nervosa

Anorexia nervosa is an eating disorder characterized by _____

self-starvation or semistarvation, sometimes to the point of death. More than 90 percent of

anorexics are _____; most are young, ambitious, and

_____ achievers. Anorexia is defined as self-starvation to the point of

weighing _____% of normal weight or having a body mass index of _____ or

less. As weight loss continues, anorexics typically lose interest in sex, become hostile and

irritable, constantly feel cold, grow a soft covering of body hair, lose scalp hair, and often

develop a preoccupation with _____. Adolescent girls are at highest risk,

but anorexia is not common. The prevalence is less than _____%, but young women

involved in dance, competitive sports, modeling, and beauty pageants are at higher risk.

Motivation of anorexics to change eating habits and to gain weight is very

_____. Forced feeding usually restores _____, but it is not a

cure. _____ behavioral therapy is more effective than most treatments but is

not used as extensively as it should be.

B. Bulimia

Bulimia is the eating disorder in which people eat huge quantities of food in an

uncontrolled manner (binge) and then get rid of the food by _____ or using

laxatives (purge). Compared with anorexics, bulimics are likely to be older, impulsive,

aware that their eating habits are _____, filled with guilt, and depressed.

Like anorexics, most bulimics are _____. Bulimia is almost never fatal, but eating large quantities of sweets can result in a deficiency of sugar in the blood called _____. Other health consequences of frequent purging include anemia, or inadequate _____ _____ cells, electrolyte imbalance, and alkalosis, an abnormally high level of alkaline in the body tissues. Unlike _____, bulimics usually have some motivation to get better.

C. Binge Eating Disorder

Binge eating disorder consists of the same out of control eating that characterizes _____, but people with binge eating disorder do not purge. Binge eating combined with *not* purging often leads to weight gain and _____. Like other eating disorders, binge eating is more common among _____, but men have this disorder more often than other eating disorders. Indeed, binge eating disorder affects at least _____% of the population. People with binge eating disorder may seek therapy, either for the binge eating or for weight problems. Cognitive behavioral therapy is effective in treating binge eating but less effective in promoting

_____ _____.

Multiple Choice Questions

_____ 1. Similar to most people who are anorexic, which of these statements was true of Mary-Kate Olsen?
   a. She has been thin throughout her entire life.
   b. She has experienced large cycles of weight gain and loss.
   c. She experienced a distorted body image.
   d. She frequently steals food and other items.

_____ 2. Which of these statements is typical of most bulimics?
   a. They are usually younger than anorexics.
   b. They exercise vigorously for long periods of time.
   c. They are usually thinner than anorexics.
   d. They use laxatives and vomiting as a means of weight control.

_____ 3. Peristalsis is
   a. the first step in the digestive process.
   b. the rhythmic contraction and relaxation of muscles that propel food through the digestive system.
   c. the exchange of gases across the alveoli.
   d. both a and b.

_____ 4. Hormones provide signals that are involved in regulating eating. The hormone _____ seems to prompt eating, and the hormone _____ produces feelings of satiation, which stops eating.
   a. leptin . . . ghrelin
   b. leptin . . . insulin
   c. insulin . . . leptin
   d. ghrelin . . . cholecystokinin

_____ 5. During World War II, a team of researchers found that normal young men changed their behavior, began to exhibit irritability and aggression, lost interest in sex and other activities, and became preoccupied with food. These young men were showing the effects of
   a. amphetamine use.
   b. living in a prison camp.
   c. experimental overfeeding.
   d. semistarvation.

_____ 6. Campbell's weight is 20 pounds below normal as a result of 2 months of a 600-calorie-a-day diet. You would expect that Campbell will
   a. feel more energetic than usual.
   b. become disinterested in food.
   c. be constantly hungry.
   d. not be able to regain his normal weight even after he increases his food intake to 3,200 calories a day.

_____ 7. Being overweight
   a. has a survival advantage during times of food shortages.
   b. greatly decreases one's energy level.
   c. is solely a matter of heredity.
   d. all of the above.

_____ 8. Ethan Allen Sims studied inmates at the Vermont State prison and found that
   a. losing weight below one's natural weight is nearly impossible.
   b. initial weight gain is easy when people consume a large number of calories, but after a high level of weight gain is achieved, additional gain is quite difficult.
   c. these prisoners were much like female anorexics.
   d. all the prisoners were able to achieve their weight goals.

_____ 9. Unlike weight charts, the waist-to-hip ratio measures
   a. the distribution of body fat.
   b. level of obesity.
   c. total weight.
   d. inheritability of obesity.

_____ 10. The definition of body mass index includes
   a. body build.
   b. age.
   c. gender.
   d. height and weight.
   e. all of the above.

_____ 11. A man 5 feet, 8 inches tall with a body mass index of 27 would weigh about _____, and a woman the same height and same body mass index would weigh about ____
   a. 145 . . . 174
   b. 174 . . . 145
   c. 213 . . . 123
   d. 134 . . . 134
   e. 177 . . . 177

_____ 12. The notion that people have a type of internal thermostat that regulates how much they weigh is called
   a. the glucostatic mechanism.
   b. the setpoint concept.
   c. adipose range.
   d. the lipostatic mechanism.

_____ 13. During the past 10 years, the people of the United States have been becoming more health conscious. At the same time,
   a. obesity rates are increasing.
   b. people are consuming fewer calories.
   c. people are consuming far more fat.
   d. both b and c.

_____ 14. Which of these statements is most consistent with the positive incentive model?
   a. People eat primarily to store calories for times when food is not plentiful.
   b. People have a biologically determined weight and will have difficulty deviating from that weight.
   c. A person who has just finished a large meal will still want to eat a luscious dessert.
   d. A person will eat huge quantities of food in an effort to resolve inner conflict.

_____15. Which of these people has the HIGHEST risk of a weight-related health problem?
    a. a 19-year-old woman whose weight is 15% above that suggested by the weight chart
    b. a middle-aged man who is 22 pounds overweight and whose weight is quite stable
    c. a middle-aged man who is 22 pounds overweight, with most of the extra pounds distributed around his middle
    d. a middle-age women who is 20 pounds overweight, with most of the extra pounds distributed around her hips and thighs

_____16. Which of these groups of people is MOST likely to diet to lose weight?
    a. adolescent boys
    b. adolescent girls
    c. African American women
    d. European American men

_____17. People wanting to lose weight should
    a. avoid physical activity because it increases appetite.
    b. avoid exercise because it raises the setpoint.
    c. incorporate exercise into their daily routine.
    d. exercise regularly and eat a high calorie diet.

_____18. People who go on low-carbohydrate diets
    a. do not lose weight.
    b. have made good nutritional choices.
    c. often experience a problem with maintaining the diet.
    d. should not include exercise as part of their routine.

_____19. Most people who are successful in losing weight
    a. follow a low-carbohydrate program.
    b. follow a low-fat program.
    c. take diet pills or have surgery.
    d. do so on their own rather than seeking professional help.

_____20. Which of these weight-related factors is the LOWEST risk for all-cause mortality for middle-aged European American women?
    a. a percent of body fat between 30% and 35%
    b. a waist-to-hip ratio of 0.72
    c. a body mass index of 40.0
    d. a history of being 30 to 35 pounds over ideal weight

_____21. When Marshall was a 21-year-old college junior, he was five feet nine inches tall and weighed 155 pounds. Now at age 60, Marshall weighs 170 pounds. Thus, Marshall
    a. is at an elevated risk for mortality due to gaining 15 pounds.
    b. should diet until he weighs about 155 to 160 pounds.
    c. should diet until he weighs less than 150 pounds.
    d. should not worry about the additional 15 pounds.
    e. both a and b.

_____22. During the past 2 decades, the average U.S. adult has decreased dietary fat from 40% of energy intake to about 33%. During this time, the average U.S. adult has
   a. become fatter.
   b. become thinner due to increased exercise.
   c. become thinner due to this reduction in dietary fat.
   d. decreased sugar intake.

_____23. In helping people lose weight, behavior modification programs
   a. reward overweight participants for each five pounds they lose.
   b. punish overweight participants if they lose weight.
   c. reward overweight participants for proper eating behaviors.
   d. punish overweight participants for improper eating behaviors.

_____24. Obese people who lose some weight but fail to attain their ideal weight
   a. have probably decreased their health risks by losing some weight.
   b. should be alarmed about this failure because they have raised rather than lowered their health risks.
   c. should try a high-fat, high-carbohydrate diet.
   d. should consider smoking as an added weight loss strategy.

_____25. Anorexics are LEAST likely to
   a. see themselves as too thin.
   b. be preoccupied with food.
   c. be ambitious and perfectionistic.
   d. have hostile feelings toward their mother.

_____26. The *DSM-IV-TR* of the American Psychiatric Association considers a person to be anorexic if that person
   a. weighs less than 100 pounds.
   b. has a waist to hip ratio of 0.80.
   c. has intentionally lost weight to 85% of the weight considered normal by the Metropolitan Life Insurance tables.
   d. has a body mass index of 18 to 25.

_____27. Which of these conditions is MOST characteristics of a person with bulimia?
   a. severely overweight
   b. severely underweight
   c. use of laxatives to purge
   d. amenorrhea

_____28. The *DSM-IV-TR* of the American Psychiatric Associations considers a person to have bulimia if that person
   a. engages in recurrent episodes of bingeing, experiences feelings of lack of control, and purges.
   b. engages in recurrent episodes of bingeing without purging.
   c. engages in purging without bingeing.
   d. all of the above.

_____29. Considering anorexia and bulimia,
   a. bulimia is more likely to be fatal.
   b. bulimics are more likely to be thinner.
   c. anorexics are more likely to be male.
   d. treatment programs for bulimia are more likely to be successful.
   e. none of the above.

_____30. What distinguishes bulimia from binge eating?
   a. Bulimics have poor impulse control, but binge eaters have better control.
   b. Bulimics restrict the amount of food they eat during a binge, but binge eaters do not.
   c. Bulimics purge, but binge eaters do not.
   d. Bulimics are likely to be overweight, but binge eaters are not.

Key Terms

Define each of the following:

anorexia nervosa —

binge eating —

BMI —

body image —

bulimia —

cholecystokinin —

ghrelin —

hypothalamus —

leptin —

peristalsis —

positive incentive model —

setpoint model —

Matching

Match the following:

1. diet pills, fasting, and purging
2. positive incentive model
3. cholecystokinin
4. small intestines
5. cardiovascular disease and diabetes
6. periods of uncontrolled eating without purging
7. anorexia nervosa
8. setpoint model
9. bulimia
10. body image problems

a. obesity increases risks

b. location of most digestion

c. binge eating disorder

d. risky dieting strategies

e. vomiting and laxative abuse

f. body mass index of 17.2

g. precursor of eating disorders

h. hunger is only one motivation for eating

i. peptide hormone that affects feelings of satiation

j. weight regulation is homeostatic

1. _____ 2. _____ 3. _____ 4. _____ 5. _____

6. _____ 7. _____ 8. _____ 9. _____ 10. _____

Essay Questions

1. Loraine is 15 pounds overweight, which is causing her to have health concerns. Loraine believes that she needs to go on a diet to lose the weight as quickly as possible. Is she correct about the health implications of her extra pounds, and what type of diet should she avoid?

2. You receive a case report of a young woman with an eating disorder, but the report does not say whether she is anorexic, bulimic, or a binge eater. What symptoms would you look for to determine which disorder she has?

Let's Get Personal—
Analyzing Your Eating

To better understand your eating patterns, keep a food diary for at least a week. Record when you eat, the types of food and beverages, and estimated portion sizes. Choose a typical week to keep your record, and try not to change your eating. Don't cheat—you won't be able to understand your eating if you make changes or fail to report honestly. The goal of keeping the food diary is to get information so that you can analyze how healthy your diet and eating patterns are.

Day 1

Breakfast   Time:

_____

_____

Snack   Time:

_____

Lunch   Time:

_____

_____

Snack   Time:

_____

Dinner   Time:

_____

Day 2

Breakfast   Time:

_____

_____

Snack   Time:

_____

Lunch   Time:

_____

_____

Snack   Time:

_____

Dinner   Time:

_____

_____

_____

Snack   Time:

_____

Day 3

Breakfast   Time:

_____

_____

_____

Snack   Time:

_____

Lunch   Time:

_____

_____

Snack   Time:

_____

Dinner   Time:

_____

_____

_____

_____

_____

Snack   Time:

_____

Day 4

Breakfast   Time:

_____

_____

_____

Snack   Time:

_____

Lunch   Time:

_____

_____

Snack   Time:

_____

Dinner   Time:

_____

_____

_____

Snack   Time: Snack   Time:

_____   _____

Day 5   **Day 6**

Breakfast   Time: Breakfast   Time:

_____   _____

_____   _____

_____   _____

Snack   Time: Snack   Time:

_____   _____

Lunch   Time: Lunch   Time:

_____   _____

_____   _____

_____   _____

Snack   Time: Snack   Time:

_____   _____

Dinner   Time: Dinner   Time:

_____   _____

_____   _____

_____   _____

Snack   Time: Snack   Time:

_____   _____

Day 7

Breakfast   Time:

_____

_____

_____

Snack   Time:

_____

Lunch   Time:

_____

_____

_____

Snack   Time:

_____

Dinner   Time:

_____

_____

_____

Snack   Time:

_____

_____

Did anything surprise you about your eating? Do you eat more than you had imagined? Do you eat more "junk foods" than you thought? Do you skip meals, either in an attempt to diet or because you have little time? Did skipping meals result in snacking or unwise choices after a skipped meal?

Answers

Fill in the Rest of the Story
I.   mouth; peristalsis; small intestine; liver; large intestine
II.   physical activity (exercise); Leptin; hypothalamus; ghrelin; cholecystokinin
II.A.   metabolism; losing; sexual; obsessed (preoccupied)
II.B.   unpleasant (difficult); difficult
III.   calories; obesity
III.A.   body fat; body mass; obesity; lowest; African; men
III.B.   setpoint; genetic; positive incentive; food
III.C.   distribution; heart (cardiovascular); middle (stomach); hips (thighs); 65
IV.   overweight; misleading; girls
IV.A.   protein; calories; reinforce (reward); exercise; medical; relapse (adherence)
IV.B.   exercising; 50; dieting
V.   bulimia
V.A.   intentional; female (women); high; 85; 17.5; food; 1; low; weight; Cognitive
V.B.   vomiting; abnormal (harmful); women; hypoglycemia; red blood; anorexics
V.C.   bulimia; obesity; women; 2; weight loss

Multiple Choice

1.	c	9	a	16.	b	24.	a
2.	d	10.	d	17.	c	25.	a
3.	b	11.	e	18.	c	26.	c
4.	d	12.	b	19.	d	27.	c
5.	d	13.	a	20.	b	28.	a
6.	c	14.	c	21.	d	29.	d
7.	a	15.	c	22.	a	30.	c
8.	b			23.	c		

Matching

1.	d	2.	h	3.	i	4.	b	5.	a
6.	c	7.	f	8.	j	9.	e	10.	g

Good points to include in your essay answers:

1. A. Loraine is probably incorrect in her belief that she needs to lose weight because of health concerns.
   1. There is a connection between obesity and several diseases, but she is not sufficiently overweight to put her at such risk.
   2. Loraine's motivation may be body image problems, which are related to the development of eating disorders.
   B. Loraine should avoid diets that
   1. Will lead to very rapid weight loss.
   2. Consist of a single food because these diets are boring, difficult to continue, and are nutritional disasters.
   3 Rely on drugs to suppress her appetite.
   4. Do not teach her healthy eating habits.

2. A. Some symptoms would not allow you to determine the difference.
   1. She would probably exhibit a great concern with weight if she had anorexia, bulimia, or binge eating disorder.
   2. She would probably be secretive about her eating habits with any of these disorders.
   B. To determine if the young woman was anorexic, bulimic, or a binge eater, you might look for
   1. Her weight—she would be (or she would desire to be) very thin if she were anorexic, her weight would most likely be normal if she were bulimic, and she would most likely be overweight if she were a binge eater.
   2. A difference in eating; anorexics refrain from eating, whereas bulimics and binge eaters both binge.
   3. Self-restraint if she were anorexic and impulsiveness if she were bulimic or a binge eater.
   4. Feelings of self-satisfaction and euphoria if she were anorexic and feelings of depression and guilt if she were bulimic or a binge eater.
   5. Dental problems that would signal bulimia but neither of the other eating disorders.
   6. A lack of willingness to be in treatment if she were anorexic and a greater willingness to be in treatment if she were bulimic or a binge eater.

272

CHAPTER 15
Exercising

Learning Objectives

After studying Chapter 15, you should be able to

1. Describe the five different types of physical activity and the benefits of each type.

2. Trace the history of research on the benefits of exercise for cardiovascular health.

3. Discuss the health benefits of exercise, including protection for specific diseases and conditions.

4. Identify the risks involved with physical activity.

5. Explain how to engage in enough but not too much physical activity to gain health benefits without excessive risks.

6. Discuss the problems of adherence to physical activity programs and provide suggestions about how to boost adherence.

Fill in the Rest of the Story

I. Types of Exercise

Nearly all types of exercise can be grouped under one of five basic kinds of physical activity, each of which may contribute to strength, flexibility, speed, or physical fitness. _____ exercise involves contracting muscles against an immovable object, which can build strength and muscle. In contrast, _____ exercise requires muscle contraction and joint movement, and this exercise also builds strength and muscle and is capable of improving body appearance. A third type of exercise, _____, requires specialized equipment that adjusts the amount of resistance according to the amount of force applied. _____ exercise involves fast, short-distance running, such as sprinting in track or running the bases in baseball. Aerobic exercise requires greatly increased _____ consumption over an extended time and can be achieved through walking, jogging, swimming, dancing, bicycling, and several other activities. Aerobic exercise benefits both the respiratory system and the

_____ system.

II. Reasons for Exercising

People who exercise list a number of reasons for exercising, including physical fitness,

weight control, and cardiorespiratory fitness.

A. Physical Fitness

Fitness can be considered either *organic* or *dynamic*. The type of fitness that refers to

inherited characteristics is called _____, whereas

_____ fitness is determined by the amount and kind of exercise a person

performs. The five basic types of exercise can contribute to muscle strength, muscle

_____, flexibility, and aerobic fitness. Of all the types of exercise, only

_____ exercise contributes to cardiovascular fitness.

B. Weight Control

Exercise combined with _____ is an excellent way to lose

weight, but exercise alone is sufficient to lower the ratio of _____ tissue to

muscle tissue and thus improve body composition. Exercise alone does not burn many

_____, but exercise performed at least four times a week does seem to

elevate _____ rate, which in turn helps control weight.

III. Cardiovascular Effects of Exercise

More important than physical fitness or weight control is the issue of exercise and

_____ health.

A. Early Studies

During the early 1950s, studies found that sedentary workers were more prone to

_____ disease than were active workers. Ralph Paffenbarger and

colleagues found that the least active Harvard graduate had a much _____

risk of heart attack. The main limitation of Paffenbarger's studies was their exclusive use of

_____ participants.

B. Later Studies

Studies over the past 25 years have tended to measure all physical activity, both on and off the _____ and to include _____ as participants. These studies have shown that a _____ lifestyle can be dangerous for women as well as for men. The Toronto Symposium looked at all available studies and found a consistent _____-_____ association between levels of physical activity and cardiovascular disease. Physical activity can help people reduce several risks, including heart disease, stroke, and _____-_____ mortality.

C. Do Women and Men Benefit Equally?

Middle-aged and older women benefit from a regular physical activity program. Moderate and vigorous activity four or five times a week yields protection against _____ _____ and all-cause mortality. Women and _____ receive similar benefits when they engage in physical activity.

D. Physical Activity and Cholesterol Levels

Aerobic exercise can raise HDL levels without raising _____-_____ lipoprotein levels, resulting in a more favorable ratio of _____ _____ to HDL. These benefits apply to a wide variety of individuals, including children and _____ as well as adults.

IV. Other Health Benefits of Physical Activity

Some evidence suggests that physical activity offers some protection against some types of cancer and _____ of bone density. In addition, exercise may be able to control diabetes and confer _____ benefits, such as decreased depression, reduced anxiety, and increased self-esteem.

A. Protection against Cancer

Regular physical activity may protect against cancer of all sites, including lung cancer, _____ cancer in women and _____ cancer in men.

B. Prevention of Bone Density Loss

Exercise can also protect women and men against _____, a disease caused by loss of calcium. Both pre- and postmenopausal women can gain protection against loss of bone density by exercise. For women and men, beginning an exercise program _____ in life and continuing throughout old age offers the most protection.

C. Control of Diabetes

Physical activity helps in the control of both _____ and _____ diabetes. Exercise is especially important in the prevention of Type 2 diabetes.

D. Psychological Benefits of Physical Activity

Research indicates that people who participate in an aerobic exercise program receive such psychological benefits as decreased depression, reduced anxiety, and _____ against stress. In general, the relationship between physical activity and psychological health is less _____ than the relationship between exercise and physical health.

Experimental studies have reported that people who engage in aerobic exercise were much _____ depressed than those who did not. Other types of exercise can also be effective. One conclusion from recent studies is that physical activity is at least as effective as _____ in dealing with depression and possibly comparable to _____ drugs.

In addition, physical activity is especially effective in reducing _____ anxiety; that is, a temporary experience of anxiety due to a specific situation. Moreover, exercise seems to buffer the negative effects of _____, but evidence is lacking that aerobic exercise can prevent stress-related illness. People who exercise regularly often have positive feelings about their body shape and physical health, which may contribute to their feelings of high

_____-_____.

V. Hazards of Physical Activity

Although its benefits are numerous, a regular physical activity program is also associated
with some potential dangers.

A. Exercise Addiction

Some people become so _____ on exercise that it interferes with
other parts of their lives, including indications such as continuing to exercise while

_____ and ignoring work and family obligations.

B. Injuries from Physical Activity

Regular exercisers are also at risk for a variety of injuries, but

_____ injury is the most common. Injuries are most frequent

among _____ exercisers, such as "weekend athletes."

C. Death during Exercise

People with preexisting heart disease should receive a _____

checkup prior to beginning program of intense physical activity because they are at

increased for death during exercise. A _____ test is a wise precaution for

older, unfit, sedentary people who want to begin an exercise program.

D. Reducing Exercise Injuries

Decreasing exercise injuries includes avoiding dangerous conditions such as pollution,

dogs, very high or low _____, and traffic. Even simple protective measures

such as choosing appropriate equipment and _____ reduces injuries.

VI. How Much Is Enough but Not Too Much?

In recent years, many experts have come to view exercise as a subset of

_____ _____, and they have emphasized the benefit of

_____ rather than prolonged or strenuous activity. Experts now recommend

that every adult should accumulate _____ minutes of moderate physical activity a day, or at least on most days. More exercise may improve endurance or body composition, but it may

also increase the risk of injuries without adding to _____ fitness.

VII. Adhering to a Physical Activity Program

Only about _____% of people in the United States meet the physical activity

requirements for health, and women do _____ than men.

A. Predicting Dropouts

A number of factors are related to exercise dropouts, including low motivation,

depression, low self-efficacy, obesity, being a smoker, having a blue collar job, and having a

_____ lifestyle. The most common reason given for quitting exercise is

_____ .

B. Increasing Maintenance

Psychological programs can increase exercise maintenance. These programs include

positive _____ for healthy behaviors, contracting, self-monitoring,

instruction, modeling, goal setting, increased self-efficacy, and _____

prevention. Another strategy for increasing physical activity is to build a more active

lifestyle rather than start on an _____ regimen.

Multiple Choice Questions

_____ 1. An example of isotonic exercise would be
   a. pushing hard against a solid wall.
   b. lifting weights.
   c. running 100 yards very quickly.
   d. jogging five miles.

_____ 2. The goal of isometric exercise is to
   a. increase cardiovascular fitness.
   b. increase muscle strength.
   c. reduce state anxiety.
   d. to increase oxygen intake.

_____ 3. An example of anaerobic exercise would be
   a. pushing hard against a solid wall.
   b. lifting weights.
   c. running 100 meters quickly.
   d. jogging five miles.

_____ 4. What type of exercise uses specialized equipment that adjusts the amount of resistance according to the amount of force applied, thus requiring exertion for lifting and additional effort for returning to the starting position?
   a. isokinetic
   b. isotonic
   c. isometric
   d. anaerobic
   e. aerobic

_____ 5. An example of aerobic exercise would be
   a. pushing hard against a sold wall.
   b. lifting weights.
   c. running 100 yards quickly.
   d. jogging five miles.

_____ 6. Randall has always wanted to be an outstanding athlete, but he has very little natural ability. Nevertheless, Randall has worked hard and is currently a distance runner at his university. Randall now has
   a. organic fitness.
   b. dynamic fitness.
   c. both of the above.
   d. neither a nor b.

_____ 7. Aerobic fitness decreases
   a. cardiorespiratory fitness.
   b. risk of heart disease.
   c. organic fitness.
   d. muscle flexibility.

_____ 8. People who lose weight through exercise do so mostly because
   a. exercise burns calories at a fast rate.
   b. exercise diminishes appetite and thus decreases food consumption.
   c. exercise elevates metabolism.
   d. they tend to diet in order to improve their appearance in exercise clothes.

_____ 9. Your friend Clayton is a sedentary, slightly overweight smoker who asks you for advice on quitting smoking. He is worried that he may gain too much weight if he quits. What advice should you give him?
   a. Quit smoking, go on a very low calorie diet, and then begin a regular physical activity program.
   b. Quit smoking, eat regularly, and begin a program of physical activity that gradually builds up to at least 3 hours a week.
   c. Quit smoking, begin a 1,000 calorie a day diet, and engage in isometric exercise 2 to 3 hours a week.
   d. Continue to smoke because some people who quit gain 40 to 50 pounds.

_____ 10. With regard to weight loss, which of the following is FALSE?
   a. Exercise alone can promote weight loss.
   b. Diet alone can promote weight loss.
   c. Weight loss can only be produced by a combination of diet and exercise.
   d. For most overweight people, the combination of diet and exercise would be most beneficial to good health.

_____ 11. The Harvard alumni study found that
   a. physical activity reduced one's risk of heart attack but did not increase length of life.
   b. exercise equivalent to jogging 20 miles per week decreased the risk of heart attack.
   c. exercise equivalent to jogging 40 miles per week decreased the risk of heart attack significantly more than jogging 20 miles per week.
   d. exercise increased length of life, but did not reduce one's risk of heart attack.

_____ 12. People exercise for a variety of reasons. Which of these reasons has the LEAST research to support claims of beneficial health?
   a. Exercise can protect against stroke.
   b. Exercise can protect against heart disease.
   c. Exercise can promote weight loss.
   d. Exercise is an effective means of quitting smoking.

_____ 13. Research evidence is strongest in support of the hypothesis that exercise protects against heart disease by
   a. increasing HDL.
   b. decreasing HDL.
   c. increasing LDL.
   d. decreasing LDL.

_____ 14. Adopting a regular program of physical activity is LEAST likely to bring about
   a. weight loss mostly around the thighs and hips.
   b. reduced chances of osteoporosis.
   c. increased dynamic fitness.
   d. a greater decrease of fat than of muscle.

_____15. For people interested in lowering their risk of heart disease,
   a. exercise is a valuable component in a program designed to lower risk factors.
   b. exercise alone is protective and allows less attention to diet and other risk factors.
   c. exercise will confer immunity against heart disease.
   d. exercise is more of a risk than a benefit.

_____16. People who diet (but not exercise) to lose weight will most likely
   a. lose both fat and lean tissue.
   b. lose more weight that people who both diet and increase their level of physical activity.
   c. lose more lean tissue than fat tissue.
   d. not be able to lose more than two or three pounds.

_____17. Evidence is strong that physical activity protects against cardiovascular disease. Additional evidence indicates that exercise protects against
   a. lung cancer.
   b. skin cancer.
   c. colon cancer.
   d. unintentional injuries.

_____18. Women ages 50 to 70 who begin an exercise program are likely to
   a. increase their risk for fractures.
   b. lose bone mineral density.
   c. develop osteoporosis.
   d. retain bone mineral density.
   e. both a and b.

_____19. Which of these statements is most accurate?
   a. Sedentary Type 1 male diabetics are three times more likely to die if they exercise regularly.
   b. Exercise can protect either men or women against Type 2 diabetes.
   c. Exercise offers some protection against early death for men but not for women.
   d. Exercise offers some protection against early death for women but not for men.

_____20 In general, a physical activity program is likely to
   a. increase depression in clinically depressed people.
   b. decrease depression to a degree that is clinically significant.
   c. increase depression but not to a statistically significant degree.
   d. decrease depression to a degree that is statistically significant.
   e. both b and d.

_____21. Research suggests that physical activity
   a. helps lower depression.
   b. is capable of decreasing anxiety.
   c. both a and b.
   d. neither a nor b.

_____22. Carney wishes to lower her high level of state anxiety. Which activity would you recommend?
a. jogging
b. relaxation training
c. transcendental meditation
d. any activity that provides a change of pace

_____23. Lee is quite dependent on exercise, running 10 to 15 miles every day and allowing running to interfere with his job and family life. You would guess that Lee
a. has a physiological addiction to running.
b. is an ex-college athlete who is trying to relive past achievements.
c. has low expectations of himself.
d. may be very concerned about his body and weight.

_____24. Research indicates that death during exercise
a. is more likely for people who are usually sedentary but who engage in occasional vigorous exercise.
b. is not possible for physically fit individuals.
c. occurs more for people who have a regular aerobic program than for people who exercise anaerobically once a week.
d. is less likely than death while watching television.

_____25. Fernando is a 24-year-old banker who is 25 pounds overweight and who wants to begin an exercise program to lose weight. You would advise him to
a. begin by jogging four or five miles a day, six days a week.
b. keep repeating to himself, "No pain, no gain."
c. weigh himself every day to document the effectiveness of his exercise program.
d. begin slowly and gradually work up to 30 minutes of moderate physical activity, 5 days a week.

_____26. Which of these people is most likely to drop out of an exercise program?
a. a married 67-year-old man who has begun a supervised exercise program as part of cardiac rehabilitation
b. a 45-year-old lawyer who has been jogging five times a week for 19 years
c. an unmarried, 32-year-old woman who is overweight and has three young children
d. a 24-year-old man who has been an avid runner for four years and who runs in spite of a series of nagging injuries

_____27. Experts currently recommend that
a. people with a history of heart problems avoid hard physical activity.
b. adults accumulate 30 minutes of moderate physical activity a day or at least on most days.
c. children benefit from moderate exercise but adults do not.
d. adults benefit from moderate exercise but children do not.

_____28. A review of 40 years of research on physical activity found that
  a. people who exercise 4 to 6 hours a week can double their protection against CVD by doubling their exercise.
  b. an inactive lifestyle is not as important a risk for CVD as high cholesterol and high blood pressure.
  c. jogging but not other forms of physical activity was protective for CVD and cancer.
  d. people who have exercised regularly for 10 or more years lose most of their protection against CVD mortality if they stop exercising for 5 or more years.

Key Terms

Define each of the following:

aerobic exercise —

anaerobic exercise —

cardiorespiratory fitness —

exercise addiction —

isokinetic exercise —

isotonic exercise —

osteoporosis —

state anxiety —

trait anxiety —

Matching

Match the following:

1. isotonic exercise

2. dose-response relationship

3. existing cardiovascular disease

4. only aerobic exercise

5. raises HDL levels

6. osteoporosis

7. behavior modification programs

8. aerobic and nonaerobic exercise

9. benefits of exercise

10. high educational and income level

a. control of diabetes and lower risk of some cancers

b. calisthenics and weight lifting

c. capable of improving exercise adherence

d. increases the chance of meeting physical activity recommendations

e. more exercise, lower all-cause mortality

f. capable of alleviating depression

g. aerobic exercise

h. hazard for sudden death during exercise

i. loss of bone mineral density

j. capable of building cardiorespiratory fitness

1. _____ 2. _____ 3. _____ 4. _____ 5. _____

6. _____ 7. _____ 8. _____ 9. _____ 10. _____

Benefits of exercise

Fill in the missing blanks to describe the benefits of physical activity.

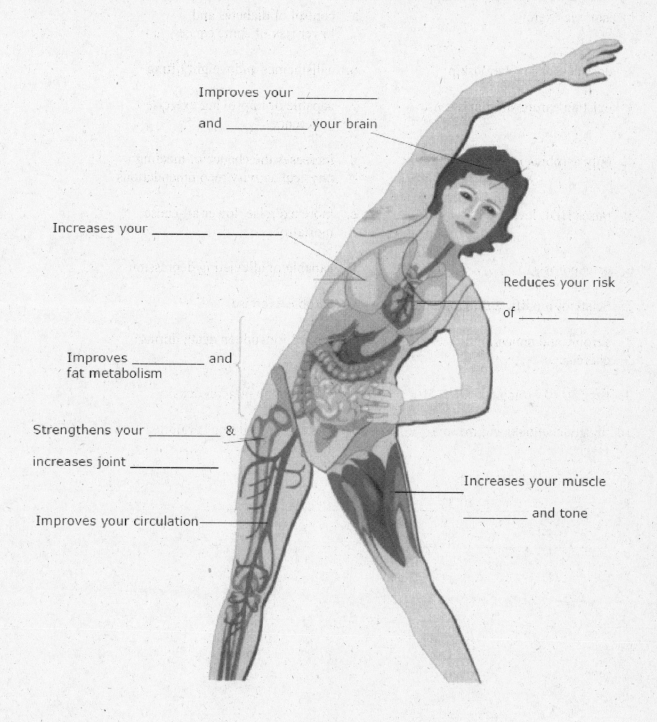

Improves your _____

and _____ your brain

Increases your _____ _____

Reduces your risk

of _____ _____

Improves _____ and
fat metabolism

Strengthens your _____ &

increases joint _____

Increases your muscle

_____ and tone

Improves your circulation

285

Essay Questions

1. Evaluate the statement, "It takes too much exercise to burn off the calories in this ice cream bar. I'd be better off just skipping the ice cream and not having to do the exercise."

2. Graham is a 45-year-old accountant who is considering beginning an exercise program to lower his chances for heart disease. Advise him about 1) types of physical activity, 2) the benefits he can expect, and 3) the hazards he needs to consider.

Let's Get Personal—
Work Out

Do you get enough exercise but not too much? Exercise too little, and you fail to gain health benefits. Exercise too much, and you risk injury. Should you play a sport, lift weights, run, do aerobics, or some combination? Determining what is the right amount and right type of exercise is not easy.

Examine your exercise habits by answering the following questions:

Do you have an exercise program?

Does your exercising best fit the pattern of

Activity at least 4 days a week

Sedentary weekdays and active weekends

Circle the type or types of exercise you perform.

Isometric   Isotonic   Isokinetic   Anaerobic   Aerobic

How long is each of your exercise sessions?

Do you exercise enough to get optimal health benefits—that is, do you expend 2,000 kcal per week in cumulative energy expenditure?

What injuries have you sustained during the past 6 months as a result of exercise?

What health benefits do you believe that you get from your exercising?

Answers

Fill in the Rest of the Story

I.   Isometric; isotonic; isokinetic; Anaerobic; oxygen; circulatory (cardiovascular)
II.A.   organic; dynamic; endurance; aerobic
II.B.   diet; fat; calories; metabolic
III.   cardiovascular
III.A. heart (cardiovascular); increased; male
III.B. job; women; sedentary (inactive); dose-response; all-cause
III.C. cardiovascular disease; men
III.D. low-density; total cholesterol; adolescents
IV.   loss; psychosocial
IV.A.   breast; prostate
IV.B.   osteoporosis; early
IV.C.   Type 1; Type 2
IV.D.   buffer; strong (clear); less; psychotherapy; antidepressant; state; stress; self-esteem
V.A.   dependent; injured
V.B.   musculoskeletal; infrequent
V.C.   medical; stress
V.D.   temperatures; clothing (shoes)
VI.   physical activity; moderate; 30; cardiovascular
VII.   25; worse
VII.A. sedentary; injury
VII.B. reinforcement; relapse; exercise

Multiple Choice

1.	b	8.	c	15	a	22.	d
2.	b	9.	b	16.	a	23.	d
3.	c	10.	c	17.	c	24.	a
4.	a	11.	b	18.	d	25.	d
5.	d	12.	d	19.	b	26.	c
6.	b	13.	a	20.	e	27.	b
7.	b	14.	a	21.	c	28.	d

Matching

1.	b	2.	e	3.	h	4.	j	5.	g
6.	i	7.	c	8.	f	9.	a	10.	d

Good points to include in your essay answers:

1. A. Exercise alone does not expend many calories BUT
   1. Exercise alone can produce weight loss.
   2. Exercise may raise the metabolic level and have an effect on weight regulation.
   B. Exercise is a beneficial component in a weight loss or weight maintenance program.
   1. Physical activity is a factor in the weight-maintenance equation, increasing the number of calories expended and building muscle tissue.
   2. Exercise can help maintain lean body mass in moderate-weight exercisers.

2. A. Graham has many choices in terms of types of exercise and physical activities.
   1. If he wants cardiovascular benefits, he needs to choose some type of aerobic exercise.
   2. Graham does not need to run or even jog; he can get aerobic benefits from walking briskly.
   3. He should exercise 5 times a week, for 30 minutes per day, and he should understand that strength training is also necessary to achieve acceptable fitness.
   B. Like almost everyone, Graham could benefit from physical activity.
   1. Research shows that aerobic exercise has cardiovascular benefits.
   2. Graham can also lower his risk of several types of cancer, improve bone mineral density, and decreases depression and anxiety through exercise.
   C. Graham also puts himself at risk by exercising.
   1. Graham should have a stress test before he begins his program; his age and lack of activity put him at risk for undetected cardiovascular disease.
   2. He needs to choose an activity and activity level that will minimize the risk for injuries.
   3. He needs to obtain the correct equipment to exercise safely.
   4. He needs to choose an environment that is safe for exercising.

CHAPTER 16
Future Challenges

Learning Objectives

After studying Chapter 16, you should be able to

1. Describe the difference between life expectancy and health expectancy.

2. Discuss the relationship of health disparities and ethnicity in the United States, including specific examples for each ethnic group.

3. Specify the progress in health psychology and the challenges facing its future.

4. Identify factors that underlie rising health care costs.

5. Critique the current health care system in the United States and offer alternatives.

6. Personalize health psychology by understanding the ways in which their behavior raises or lowers their health risks.

7. Describe some healthy lifestyle choices that they can adopt now to decrease future risks.

Fill in the Rest of the Story

I. Healthier People

Americans are inundated with health information, and this knowledge has been translated into

action in some ways because the mortality rate has declined for cardiovascular disease,

_____, and unintentional injuries. National policy is reflected in *Healthy*

People 2010, a report that sets both broad and specific goals. The broad goals include increasing the

span of _____ life and reducing health disparities among Americans.

A. Increasing the Span of Healthy Life

Increasing the span of healthy life is different from increasing life

_____. A healthy life means being free from dysfunction, disease

symptoms, and health-related problems. Each year of healthy life is called a

_____ year. Health _____ is the period of life people spend free from disability.

B. Reducing Health Disparities

The United States does a _____ job of dispensing health care to its citizens than any other industrialized nation. African Americans, Hispanic Americans, and _____ Americans have lower income and educational levels than European Americans and _____ Americans. These income disparities relate to lower educational levels, which produces lower _____ literacy. Individuals with low health literacy tend to have poorer access to health services, more risky behaviors, fewer health-protective behaviors, and shorter _____ _____.

II. Outlook for Health Psychology

Despite rapid growth, health psychology faces challenges for its future.

A. Progress in Health Psychology

Health psychology showed rapid growth and changed the mission statement of psychology to include issues related to physical _____. The progress included a growing body of _____ and applications to provide care and _____ to individuals.

B. Future Challenges for Health Care

Two important challenges that health psychology must meet are the changing profile of _____ and the escalation of _____ _____ costs. The population of the United States and most other industrialized countries is aging, which means that health care systems will be faced with a growing need for health care for _____ diseases. An additional challenge for health psychology is the rising costs of health care, which have increased at a much higher rate than _____.

C. Will Health Psychology Continue to Grow?

Health psychologists' commitment to the biopsychosocial model has helped to promote a comprehensive view of health and has striven to end the false dichotomy between mental and _____ health. With their expertise firmly established, clinical health psychologists have moved into a variety of settings, and some are training to be _____ health care providers.

III. Making Health Psychology Personal

The volume of research in health psychology can provide guidelines for individuals to personalize health psychology by making changes in their behavior to improve their _____.

A. Understanding Your Risks

College students see their health as good to excellent, and that perception is typically _____. However, that perception may lead young people to believe that they are not _____ to health problems, which is not accurate. College students are unlikely to show signs of heart disease but are most vulnerable to _____ injuries and violence. Of these injuries, _____ crashes are the most common source of injury and death for young people, and _____ is often involved. Indeed, college students are more likely than others the same age to _____ after drinking. Adolescence and young adulthood is also a time during which individuals adopt lifestyles that may either _____ to or protect against health risks.

B. Cultivating a Healthy Lifestyle

The huge amount of health information that people receive may not help them make good choices. People often lack the _____ _____ to evaluate this abundance of information. Relying on findings from the Alameda County Study, good behaviors to

adopt include avoiding _____, engaging in regular physical _____,

drinking alcohol in moderation or not at all, maintaining a healthy weight, and getting 7 to 8

hours of _____ per night. People who practice these behaviors live a

_____, healthier life.

Multiple Choice Questions

_____ 1. During the past 35 years, the people of the United States have
   a. increased the amount of saturated fat in their diets.
   b. increased their rate of death from unintentional injuries.
   c. decreased their use of seatbelts and airbags.
   d. decreased their rate of cardiovascular disease.

_____ 2. Over the past 10 years, death rates in the in the United States for _____ have been declining.
   a. cardiovascular disease
   b. cancer
   c. homicide
   d. unintentional injuries
   e. all of the above

_____ 3. *Healthy People 2010* set two primary goals for the people of the United States. One is to eliminate health disparities, and the second is to
   a. reduce the rate of deaths from cardiovascular disease.
   b. discover the causes of Alzheimer's disease.
   c. increase the quality and years of healthy life.
   d. find a cure for cancer.

_____ 4. At age 65, women in the United States have another 19 years of life expectancy and about _____ years of health expectancy.
   a. 5
   b. 10
   c. 15
   d. 22

_____ 5. Compared with other industrialized countries, the United States ranks _____ in dispensing health care to its citizens.
   a. first
   b. third
   c. seventh
   d. last

_____ 6. In the United States, wealthy people, compared with poor people,
   a. have a shorter life expectancy.
   b. have more years of healthy life.
   c. have more heart disease but no more deaths from heart disease.
   d. have more deaths from heart disease but similar rates of heart disease.

_____ 7. Compared with African Americans, European Americans have
   a. a longer life expectancy.
   b. a higher infant mortality rate.
   c. an increased risk of death from cardiovascular disease.
   d. an increased risk of death from homicide.

_____ 8. Among Hispanic Americans, which people have the most education and the greatest likelihood of adequate health care and physician visits?
   a. Haitian Americans
   b. Puerto Rican Americans
   c. Mexican Americans
   d. Cuban Americans

_____ 9. Socioeconomic status has a strong influence on receiving health care in the United States. However, when socioeconomic factors are adjusted, which group has a high rate of risky behaviors and a low rate of receiving health services?
   a. Cuban Americans
   b. Asian Americans
   c. Native Americans
   d. European Americans

_____ 10. Which group has the longest life expectancy and the best health of any ethnic group in the United States?
   a. Asian Americans
   b. European Americans
   c. Native Americans
   d. Mexican Americans

_____ 11. For at least 2,000 years, some people have been advocating moderation in all things. This seems to be good advice for about every health-related behavior except
   a. eating candy.
   b. exercising.
   c. drinking alcohol.
   d. smoking cigarettes.

_____12. An example of secondary prevention would be
   a. early screening of people at risk for breast cancer.
   b. smoking prevention programs in elementary schools.
   c. improving the training of physicians, nurses, and other medical personnel.
   d. treating cancer patients with chemotherapy.

_____13. At what point in a person's life will adopting a healthy lifestyle produce health benefits?
   a. A healthy lifestyle will produce benefits only if the person begins during adolescence.
   b. A healthy lifestyle will be beneficial if adopted by age 35 but not later.
   c. A person may be middle-aged and still receive benefits from adopting a healthy lifestyle.
   d. A person may receive health benefits by adopting healthy behaviors even at age 65.

_____14. Which of these is NOT a major factor in the increasing costs of health care in the United States?
   a. increase in number of HMOs
   b. too many hospitals and hospital beds
   c. specialization among physicians
   d. inefficient administration of health services

_____15. College students who perceive their health as excellent and believe that it will remain so
   a. may ignore the risks posed by their behavior.
   b. usually adopt healthy habits to maintain their good health.
   c. often use avoidant coping strategies such as drinking alcohol.
   d. are more likely to be female than male.

_____16. A majority of deaths among college students can be attributed to
   a. risky behaviors that contribute to unintentional injuries.
   b. an unhealthy diet.
   c. smoking.
   d. homicide and suicide.

_____17. Which of the following risky behaviors is more common among college students than others in the same age group?
   a. smoking cigarettes
   b. driving after drinking
   c. eating a high-carbohydrate diet
   d. getting less than four hours of sleep a night

_____18. One health advantage college students have over those who do not attend college is that
   a. they are less likely to smoke cigarettes.
   b. they are less likely to binge drink.
   c. they are less likely to drive after drinking.
   d. both b and c.
   e. all of the above.

Key Terms

Define each of the following:

Boulder model —

health disparities —

health expectancy —

primary prevention —

secondary prevention —

well-year —

Matching

Match the following:

1. automobile crashes

2. acceptance by health care professionals

3. goal of *Healthy People 2010*

4. worse at dispensing health care than any industrialized country

5. shortest life expectancy of any ethnic group in U. S.

6. longest life expectancy of any ethnic group in U. S.

7. a year free of dysfunction

8. binge drinking

9. insurance coverage

a. critical factor for growth of health psychology

b. United States

c. well year

d. Native Americans

e. Asian Americans

f. increasing the span of healthy life

g. health risk more common among college students

h. leading cause of death for college students

i. access to health care

1. _____ 2. _____ 3. _____ 4. _____ 5. _____

6. _____ 7. _____ 8. _____ 9. _____

Where Health Care Dollars Go

Divide the dollar bill and label where health care dollars go. That is, what percent of each health care dollar spent goes to physicians, hospitals, prescription drugs, and so forth?

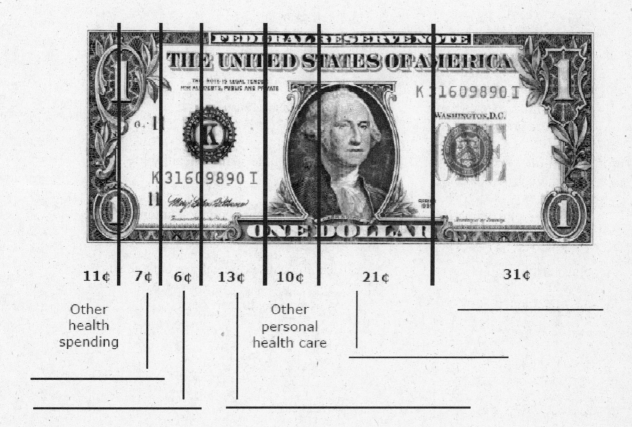

11¢   7¢   6¢   13¢   10¢   21¢   31¢

Other
health
spending

Other
personal
health care

299

Essay Questions

1. A friend of yours (who is a psychology major but who has not taken health psychology) tells you that the key to improving the health of people in the United States is through changing health-related behaviors such as alcohol and drug abuse and smoking. According to *Healthy People 2010*, is your friend correct?

2. If you wanted to adopt a healthier lifestyle based on results from health research, what behaviors would be your focus?

Let's Get Personal—
How Long a Life?

Life expectancy has increased significantly over the past 100 years, and one of the most prominent trends in health is the growth of the number of elderly. Do you think that you will be among them? How old do you think you will live to be?

After you make this estimate, compare it to the estimate you make based on the completion of an assessment you can find online. This assessment appears at http://www.livingto100.com. This assessment asks a series of questions about lifestyle and health habits as well as family background. The quiz immediately delivers a life expectancy estimate, along with a rationale for each of the questions. You can see how your behavior alters your life expectancy through adding years for good health habits and subtracting years for risky behaviors. According to this estimate, how old will you live to be?

According to this assessment, was your first estimate too optimistic or too pessimistic?

Answers

Fill in the Rest of the Story

I.   cancer; healthy
I.A.   expectancy; well; expectancy
I.B.   poorer; Native; Asian; health; life expectancy
II.A.   health; research; treatment
II.B.   illness; heath care; chronic; inflation
II.C.   physical; primary
III.   health
III.A.   correct (accurate); vulnerable; unintentional (accidental); automobile; alcohol; drive; contribute
III.B.   health literacy; smoking, activity, sleep, longer

Multiple Choice

1.	d	10.	a
2.	e	11.	d
3.	c	12.	a
4.	b	13.	d
5.	d	14.	a
6.	b	15.	a
7.	a	16.	a
8.	d	17.	b
9.	c	18.	a

Matching

1.	h	2.	a	3.	f	4.	b	5.	d
6.	e	7.	c	8.	g	9.	i		

303

Good points to include in your essay answer:

1. A. According to *Healthy People 2010*, your friend is partially (but not completely) correct. Reducing health disparities will depend on two strategies.
   B. One strategy is changing poor health habits.
   1. Many people engage in behaviors that affect their health, such as smoking, poor dietary choices, alcohol and drug abuse, and a sedentary lifestyle.
   2. These health-compromising behaviors are associated with lower educational and income levels, which is more common for African Americans, Hispanic Americans, and Native Americans than for European Americans and Asian Americans.
   C. Another strategy is reducing disparities in access to health services.
   1. People without health insurance often have limited access to health services.
   2. Limited access to health care results in failures in prevention and delays in treatment, with consequences for poor health and decreased life expectancy.

2. A. The Alameda County Study furnished results that can direct individuals to make healthy changes in behavior
   B. Cultivating five behaviors will increase life expectancy and decrease the risk for a variety of diseases.
   1. Eliminate smoking and the use of tobacco products.
   2. Engage in regular physical activity.
   3. Drink alcohol in moderation or not at all.
   4. Maintain a healthy weight.
   5. Get 7 to 8 hours of sleep a night.
   C. In addition to these five behaviors, cultivating a social support network is related to good health.